MAKING MENTAL HEALTH

Making Mental Health: A Critical History historicises mental health by examining the concept from the 'madness' of the late nineteenth century to the changing ideas about its contemporary concerns and status. It argues that a critical approach to the history of psychiatry and mental health shows them to constitute a dual clinical–political project that gathered pace over the course of the twentieth century and continues to resonate in the present. Drawing on scholarship across several areas of historical inquiry as well as historical and contemporary clinical literature, the book uses a thematic approach to highlight decisive moments that demonstrate the stakes of this engagement in Anglo-American contexts.

By tracing the (unfinished) history of institutions, the search for cures for psychiatric distress, the growing interest of the nation state in mental health, the history of attempts to globalise psychiatry, the controversies over the politics of diagnostic categories that erupted in the 1960s and 1970s, and the history of theorising about the relationship between the psyche and the market, the book offers a comprehensive account of the evolution of mental health into a commonplace concern.

Addressing key questions in the fields of history, medical humanities, and the social sciences, as well as in the psychiatry disciplines themselves, the book is an essential contribution to an ongoing conversation about mental distress and its meanings.

Elizabeth Roberts-Pedersen is a Senior Lecturer in History at the University of Newcastle, Australia. Her research examines the history of psychiatry and medicine as well as the history of warfare. Between 2016 and 2021 she was an Australian Research Council DECRA Fellow in the university's Centre for the Study of Violence.

Critical Approaches to Health

Series Editors: Kerry Chamberlain & Antonia Lyons

The Routledge *Critical Approaches to Health* series aims to present critical, interdisciplinary books around psychological, social and cultural issues related to health. Each volume in the series provides a critical approach to a particular issue or important topic, and is of interest and relevance to students and practitioners across the social sciences. The series is produced in association with the International Society of Critical Health Psychology (ISCHP).

Titles in the series:

Migration and Health
Critical Perspectives
Heide Castañeda

Rethinking Global Health
Frameworks of Power
Rochelle A. Burgess

Medical Humanities
Ethics, Aesthetics, Politics
Alan Bleakley

Making Mental Health
A Critical History
Elizabeth Roberts-Pedersen

For more information about this series, please visit: www.routledge.com/Critical-Approaches-to-Health/book-series/CRITHEA

MAKING MENTAL HEALTH

A Critical History

Elizabeth Roberts-Pedersen

Routledge
Taylor & Francis Group
LONDON AND NEW YORK

Designed cover image: Getty Images

First published 2025
by Routledge
4 Park Square, Milton Park, Abingdon, Oxon OX14 4RN

and by Routledge
605 Third Avenue, New York, NY 10158

Routledge is an imprint of the Taylor & Francis Group, an informa business

The electronic version of this book was funded to publish Open Access through Taylor & Francis' Pledge to Open, a collaborative funding open access books initiative. The full list of pledging institutions can be found on the Taylor & Francis Pledge to Open webpage.

British Library Cataloguing-in-Publication Data
A catalogue record for this book is available from the British Library

ISBN: 978-0-367-36784-8 (hbk)
ISBN: 978-0-367-36785-5 (pbk)
ISBN: 978-0-429-35146-4 (ebk)

DOI: 10.4324/9780429351464

Typeset in Times New Roman
by Apex CoVantage, LLC

CONTENTS

SERIES EDITOR PREFACE

Critical approaches to health

Health is a major issue for people all around the world and is fundamental to individual wellbeing, personal achievements, and satisfaction, as well as to families, communities, and societies. It is also embedded in social notions of participation and citizenship. Much has been written about health, from a variety of perspectives and disciplines, but a lot of this writing takes a biomedical and positivist approach to health matters, neglecting the historical, social, and cultural contexts and environments within which health is experienced, understood, and practiced. We developed this series of books to offer critical, social science perspectives on important, relevant, and timely health topics.

The *Critical Approaches to Health* series provides new writing on health by presenting books offering critical, interdisciplinary, and theoretical writing about health, where matters of health are framed quite broadly. The series seeks to include books that range across important health matters, including general health-related issues (such as gender and media), major social issues for health (such as medicalisation, obesity, and palliative care), particular health concerns (such as pain, doctor–patient interaction, health services, and health technologies), particular health problems (such as diabetes, autoimmune disease, and medically unexplained illness), or health for specific groups of people (such as the health of migrants, the homeless, and the aged), or combinations of these.

The series seeks above all to promote critical thought about health matters. By critical, we mean going beyond the critique of the topic and work in the field, to more general considerations of power and benefit, and in particular, to addressing concerns about whose understandings and interests are upheld and whose are marginalised by the approaches, findings, and practices in these various domains of health. Such critical agendas involve reflections on what constitutes knowledge, how it is created, and how it is used. Accordingly, critical approaches consider epistemological and theoretical positioning, as well as issues of methodology and practice, and seek to examine how health is enmeshed within broader social relations and structures. Books within this series take up this challenge and seek to provide new insights and understandings by applying a critical agenda to their topics. Explore the previous sixteen books in the series at *www.routledge.com/Critical-Approaches-to-Health/book-series/CRITHEA*.

In this book, *Making Mental Health: A Critical History*, Elizabeth Roberts-Pedersen takes a critical historical look at mental health, offering us a new and distinctive approach to the topic. In a wide-ranging coverage, she explores how mental health has been shaped historically over the past 150 years by the discipline of psychiatry and the inter-related histories of psychology, psychoanalysis, and related 'psy' disciplines in Western societies. She considers the various entanglements of psychiatry with adjacent disciplines that are involved in the biomedicalisation, professionalisation, and 'scientification' of psychiatry, and how together these have contributed to previous understandings of mental health disorders and their treatments. She also provides scholarly insights into how contemporary understandings of mental health are shaped by the histories of neurology and the neurosciences, as well as historical and current clinical literature.

The book is cleverly organised around a set of 'themes,' focussing on significant historical moments that are discussed in depth to reveal how mental health is 'produced' and shaped by various historical-social-political pressures. Through this organisation, Roberts-Pedersen outlines the move from mental hygiene to mental health, the changing role played by asylums, the changing nature of patient agency over time, the problematics of subjective diagnoses, the influence of the psy-complex, the reframing of the brain as biocultural, and the broader issues of race, culture, gender, as well as capitalism and the state.

The essential premise of this book is to argue for a critical approach to the history of psychiatry and mental health that positions these as dual endeavours, that is, as both clinical undertakings and as projects that have distinct political effects. Consequently, the book does not attempt to offer a definitive history of psychiatry and mental health, but rather to contribute a wider critical history that highlights important and decisive historical moments. These moments are thoughtfully chosen to reveal the stakes involved in the clinical–political intersections between psychiatry and mental health in Anglo-American contexts and to open discussion on the political entanglements and influences between them. Its penetrating and critical historical analysis of the socio-political forces that have shaped contemporary understandings and practices both in and on mental health makes the scope of this book wide-ranging, and its content challenging and provocative. The accessible writing style makes it an engaging, compelling read. It is a great addition to the *Critical Approaches to Health* series, deserving of wide readership.

Kerry Chamberlain and Antonia Lyons

ACKNOWLEDGEMENTS

My thanks, first and foremost, to series editors Kerry Chamberlain and Antonia Lyons, and to Lucy Kennedy at Routledge, for their support of this project. I'm also grateful for the encouragement and interest of my colleagues at the University of Newcastle. Special thanks go to Cathy Coleborne and Robyn Dunlop for their expert feedback on portions of the manuscript and to Kath McPhillips, Nancy Cushing, Effie Karageorgos, and Kate Ariotti for the camaraderie of our weekly writing circle. Thanks, too, to Matthew Sidebotham for his exacting attention to the reference list at a crucial juncture, and to Janet Hillis, for tolerating book talk during long runs at dawn.

I thank the State Library of New South Wales for permission to consult the Neville Yeomans papers cited in Chapter 1. Portions of Elizabeth Roberts-Pedersen, 'Towards a (bio)cultural history of the brain?', *History Australia* 19 (2022), 151–160, copyright © Australian Historical Association, appear in Chapter 2 with the permission of Informa UK Limited, trading as Taylor & Francis Group, www.tandfonline.com, on behalf of the Australian Historical Association. Research for this book was supported by Australian Research Council DECRA Fellowship DE160100623.

Finally, my love and thanks to Allan Roberts, Jill Roberts, and David Roberts for their immense practical support and ever-sensible advice, and to Naia Pedersen, Kit Pedersen, and James Pedersen - for everything.

INTRODUCTION

In the late 1980s, a historian searching for documents related to the history of the Bethlem Hospital (also known as London's infamous 'Bedlam' asylum) was alerted to the existence of a 'nondescript' leather notebook, preserved for centuries in a family collection, its covers secured with a brass clip, and small enough to slip into a pocket.[1] This was the 1766 casebook of Dr John Monro, born in 1715 and, like his father James before him and his son Thomas after him, the official physician of Bethlem from 1752 until his death in 1791.[2] In discharge of his official duties Monro visited the hospital several times a week, including on Saturdays, when he reviewed the new admissions. Yet as his surviving casebook demonstrates, he also had a lucrative private practice attending to mostly moneyed patients in their own homes or in the various private madhouses dotted throughout London—family-run establishments with which Monro often had ongoing commercial relationships.[3] As the historians Jonathan Andrews and Andrew Scull emphasise in a meticulous commentary accompanying the published edition, this document is unique. Whereas other eighteenth-century casebooks record the vicissitudes of general practice and thus illuminate mental troubles only incidentally, the one hundred cases Monro recorded between January and November 1766 provide a singular view into eighteenth-century 'mad doctoring' and the various forms of mental distress experienced by the people of the metropolis.[4]

The behaviours, symptoms, and circumstances that brought patients into contact with Monro were diverse. As Andrews and Scull suggest, unless the 1766 casebook is an aberration, historians' habitual interest in the more spectacular manifestations of 'madness'—the 'extreme case of the violent maniac or the suicidal melancholic'—risks distorting our understanding of the management of mental disorder in the eighteenth century.[5] The world of the casebook is more quotidian, with Monro's patients a mix of the nervously afflicted and those suffering from more

DOI: 10.4324/9780429351464-1

evident 'madness,' with the latter designation usually turning on patients' unruly, 'outragious,' or 'extravagant' behaviour. A Mr Mitchell, who lived 'near the Turnpike at Westminster,' was described by Monro as 'exceeding mad' on account of his 'spitting, sulky, saying nothing tumbling & tossing about, grinning, & obstinate refusing to eat, & obliged to be tied down in his bed.'[6] A Mr Hudson, who was confined to Mr Miles' madhouse, was recorded by Monro as 'extremely mad & raving at times,' so that his 'complaint has the appearance of frenzy.'[7] The 'raving' Mrs Dibsdale had to be held down.[8] Other patients, however, troubled by 'low spirits,' distressing thoughts, and poor sleep, appeared to suffer from something closer to George Cheyne's 'English malady,' a contemporaneous catch-all for nervous disturbance.[9] A Mrs Harris was 'troubled with bad & blasphemous thoughts which kept her from sleeping & made her very uneasy & unhappy.'[10] A Miss Compton in Argyle Street thought herself 'more than ordinarily wicked,' heard voices, and 'sleeps but little.'[11] An unnamed servant maid who consulted Monro about her 'low melancholy' believed 'she had not been righteous enough,' causing her to suffer from 'wicked thoughts which hinder'd her from sleeping, & kept in hurries & at some times put her quite into agonies.'[12] An anonymous patient who saw Monro in January thought himself 'low spirited' due to excessive masturbation as a young man. As with patients deemed mad, the most serious cases of such 'low melancholy' could also result in confinement. Monro saw a Mrs Cookson at Mr Duffield's madhouse, where she was 'troubled with blasphemous thoughts' and slept badly.[13] Mr Hamilton, a 'Scotch gentleman' suffering from 'an excessive depression of spirits without reason' who had made past attempts to harm himself, was confined in Mr Clarke's establishment until he could be chaperoned home.[14]

Monro's casebook is also valuable for the light it shines on therapeutics—or, more precisely, their absence. Like his peers, Monro was decidedly 'non-interventionist' and, in keeping with his gentlemanly status, literally 'hands off.'[15] The casebook's single reference to the 'blooding' of a patient suggests that Bethlem's standard program of purging, bleeding, and hot and cold bathing was less central to private practice.[16] Instead, Monro's primary function was consultative: observing the patient, occasionally making recommendations regarding confinement, and then simply waiting to see what transpired.[17] He also offered practical advice. In the first months of 1766, for example, the doctor had several encounters with a clerk whom he judged 'the most particular case of Lunacy, in the true sense of the word, I ever remember.'[18] This man complained that 'he is generally afflicted either at the new moon or the full with a kind of stupidity & dejection of spirits which makes [him] quite unfit for business,' with the onset signalled by 'an uneasiness or pain in his head,' especially when asleep with his head 'declined.'[19] In April, as the full moon approached, Monro offered the pragmatic advice to 'sleep in an easy chair & in an erect posture.' The clerk 'did so for two nights & had no return.'[20]

I begin this study of the history of mental health with Monro's casebook because as other commentators have remarked, despite the gulf of centuries it displays evocative similarities with the more recent history of psychiatry, that modern heir of mad-doctoring, and the notion of mental health it underwrites.[21] In the casebook, both 'mad' patients and patients with 'low melancholy,' obsessive thoughts, insomnia, and anxious 'hurries' inhabit a diagnostic borderland in which sanity and insanity overlap, in which periods of illness shade into periods of health and back again, where labels do not neatly contain the varieties of patients' distress nor reliably portend their outcome, where practitioners like Monro toiled in the absence of reliable therapeutics, and where confinement loomed as a final recourse. In this book, I argue that these same conceptual uncertainties have troubled psychiatry since its inception in the mid-nineteenth century, and that they continue to complicate the broader field of mental health that emerged from this discipline. In addition, I suggest that the history of psychiatry and mental health reveals them to be intertwined in a dual clinical–political project that gathered pace over the course of the twentieth century as the swiftly professionalising field of psychiatry became useful to modern states' projects of public health and broader governance. Drawing on scholarship across several areas of historical inquiry—primarily the history of psychiatry, but also the related histories of psychology, psychoanalysis and related 'psy' disciplines, and the history of neurology and the neurosciences—as well as historical and contemporary clinical literature, I use a thematic approach to highlight decisive moments that demonstrate the stakes of this clinical–political intersection in Anglo-American contexts, including in the colonial world and the Australian setting from which I write. While not intended to be a definitive history of psychiatry and mental health, the book contributes to a wider critical history of these endeavours by emphasising their political entanglements and effects.

While I locate the beginnings of a political concern with psychiatry and mental health in the mid-nineteenth century with the professionalisation and concomitant 'scientification' of psychiatry, the latter concept was not commonplace until after the Second World War. Prior to this conflict, it was used somewhat sparingly but also interchangeably with the term 'mental hygiene,' the slogan of a movement with eugenicist tendencies that garnered significant attention from clinicians, policymakers, and the public during the period between the world wars. Prior to that sparse references to 'mental health' can be found in leading Anglophone medical journals at the turn of the century and suggest that the term was understood to refer to mental or nervous trouble. In January 1902, for example, the British *Journal of Mental Science* published 'The National Mental Health and the War,' a commentary on the apparently diminishing rates of insanity admissions to asylums despite the ongoing South African War (circumstances commonly thought to increase mental agitation).[22] Another early example is a July 1906 editorial in the *Journal of the American Medical Association* titled 'Mental Health of School Children,' warning family doctors to be alert for the signs of mental strain on school-age children, the result of the 'modern overstrenuosity of education' on the 'developing brain.'[23]

References to mental health in the medical press increased after the First World War, an escalation reflecting the growing popularity of the mental hygiene movement in Anglo-American contexts, as well as the impact of that conflict on psychiatry and theories of mental distress more generally. The mental hygiene movement was closely associated with the American activist Clifford Beers, a former asylum patient and author of the bestselling *A Mind That Found Itself* (1908), an account of his ill-treatment in several psychiatric hospitals.[24] In a formulation characteristic of the many critics of the asylum, Beers argued that these institutions were as likely to make people sick as to cure them, a paradox in which 'the treatment often meted out to insane persons is the very treatment which would deprive some sane persons of their reason.'[25] An articulate Yale alumnus, Beers was a reassuring representative of the formerly insane, someone who embodied the possibility of recovery. His influential supporters included the psychologist William James and, crucially, the Swiss-American psychiatrist Adolf Meyer, the soon-to-be head of the new Phipps Psychiatric Clinic at the Johns Hopkins Hospital in Baltimore, an institution focused on preventing mental illness rather than simply treating it.[26]

In 1909, Meyer and Beers co-founded the National Committee for Mental Hygiene, an organisation with an encompassing mandate that soon diverged from the welfare of institutionalised patients towards the identification and prevention of mental disorders in the community at large. In this regard, Meyer's 'psychobiological' approach to psychiatric illness—attentive to all factors that might cause individual cases of mental disorder, open to various forms of intervention, but agnostic as to ultimate causes—was critical to this widened scope. While Meyer's formulations were notoriously opaque, his governing conceit was simple: mental health was a state of 'equilibrium,' whereas mental illness was a form of 'dissolution' or maladjustment. And, because the genesis of mental illness was multifactorial—not just hereditarian but also environmental and circumstantial—it was possible not just to treat mental disorders but to intervene to prevent them.[27] A resulting ethos of early intervention fostered the establishment of mental hygiene clinics in major cities during the interwar period, a development aided by the expansion of the psychiatric workforce to include other professions, such as psychiatric social workers, occupational therapists, and clinical psychologists.[28] Mental hygiene also implied the need to scrutinise the emotional stability and intelligence of children and in the interwar period, the growing number of references to 'mental health' in the medical press often related to childhood. The book review section of the *Journal of the American Medical Association*, for example, often featured primers on children's mental health.[29] In interwar British publications, the term was also associated with child development as well as the mental status of the population at large.[30] It was also reflected in administrative reform. The Board of Control, the body governing the treatment of the mentally ill in Britain, adopted the term during the 1920s.[31] The renaming of the British journal *Mental Welfare* as *Mental Health* in 1940, in anticipation of the final recommendations of the Feversham Committee regarding greater coordination of services for mental disorders and mental deficiency, was emblematic.[32] The final issue of *Mental Welfare* reproduced a speech by Sir Laurence Brock, chair of the Board of Control, in which he presented mental health as a broad area of official concern, suggesting that there was no hard line between sanity and insanity, and that mental health services required greater centralisation and a larger focus on prevention.[33]

During the Second World War, the term 'mental health' became more routine, and by the end of the conflict, it was the preferred term over 'mental hygiene,' not least because the latter, with its eugenicist links, had uncomfortable parallels with Nazi racial medicine. It also reflected the newly expanded interest by states in population health and its political implications. Immediately following the war, the term was given official imprimatur in Britain by bodies like the National Association for Mental Health (NAMH), founded in 1946, and, in the United States, by the *National Mental Health Act* (1946) and the National Institute of Mental Health, founded in 1949. It was also a key part of the agenda of the newly established World Health Organization (WHO), as I discuss in Chapter 4. Hence, by the end of the 1940s, mental health had supplanted mental hygiene, though there was ongoing disagreement over its meaning, scope, and policy implications.[34] The opening lines of an influential account published in 1958, for example, declared that '[t]here is hardly a term in current psychological thought as vague, elusive, and ambiguous as the term "mental health".' Later in the book, the author opined that mental health risked 'becoming a popular movement that lives by slogans and presents ten easy rules for being mentally healthy ever after.'[35]

In addition to the diffusion of the term 'mental health,' three strands in the history of psychiatry and its associated historiography help contextualise the political implications of clinical developments. The first relates to the asylum. As will become evident in Chapter 1, historians of psychiatry have focused much of their attention on institutional psychiatry—that is, on psychiatry as practised in asylums, madhouses, and other custodial institutions. This is logical given one of psychiatry's signal characteristics is its power to detain patients based on what the clinician believes are aberrant beliefs and behaviours.[36] The lives of institutionalised patients, the practices of institutions themselves, and the professional lives of the doctors who administered these institutions remain important for comprehending the application of psychiatric theory and practice to chronically ill patients. But as Monro's casebook suggests, we miss something fundamental if we focus solely on the asylum and the confinement of the 'mad.' Especially during the twentieth century, psychiatry changed very profoundly from a set of theories and practices closely identified with institutions and the institutionalised 'insane' to a medical science in which various kinds of practitioners—psychiatrists, psychologists, social workers, and general practitioners—now participate. This protean, 'liquid' character of psychiatry helped facilitate the expansive and diffuse character of contemporary 'mental health,' as well as reorient the relationship between clinicians and patients.[37]

The second development concerns the status of the patient directly. In 1985, the distinguished historian of medicine and psychiatry Roy Porter published a seminal article in which he took issue with the 'physician-centred' approach of much medical history.[38] For Porter, the focus on doctors risked underestimating the impact of patient agency in shaping the medical cultures of the past. He thus encouraged his fellow historians to find 'the patient's view' by reconstructing what were, after all, 'two-way encounters between doctors and patients.' In addition to shifting focus away from physicians, such a 'people's history of health' would also counter what Porter regarded as the generalising tendencies of the Foucauldian 'medicalisation' thesis, in which patients (who Porter refers to as 'sufferers') were always and forever oppressed by physicians and the broader medical establishment. Rather, for Porter, the history of medicine suggested that 'initiatives have often come from, and power has frequently rested with the sufferer, or with lay people in general, rather than with the individual physician or the medical profession at large.' Using the diarist Samuel Pepys as an example, Porter argued that in the early modern period, patients had substantial agency within the complex medical marketplace that comprised both folklore and more conventional medicine. Yet Porter's implication was that this agency might extend beyond the early modern period to patients more broadly.

While Porter's thesis risked overgeneralisation (as several historians have pointed out, Pepys' detailed diaries are hardly representative of the kinds of sources historians have readily to hand), his broader point that the history of medicine is incomplete without a corresponding, if not complementary, history of the patient, is an important one.[39] It is particularly pertinent for the history of psychiatry, where so much rests on the texture of patient–clinicians interactions but, equally, so much evidence is produced by practitioners *about* patients, and where grasping the dynamics of encounters that occurred in a wide variety of institutional and private contexts is central to understanding the history of diagnostic and therapeutic practices, as well as the lifeworlds of patients. Yet obtaining this history is difficult. Patient autobiographies and oral history interviews necessarily privilege the literate or the otherwise articulate, and documents stemming from clinicians and other medical authorities inevitably filter the patient through the medical gaze.[40] Reading the case notes of clinicians like Monro and other kinds of medical records 'against the grain' is one technique here, and scholars continue to find and trial new sources and methods to reveal the experience of patients.[41] Still, patients are all too often elusive figures, always in danger of slipping from view. In this book, too, while I have tried to illuminate the general effects of changes in psychiatric theory and practice on patients, I am conscious that this risks rendering them the narrow objects of psychiatry, rather than actors in their own right. The mad activist movement, discussed in Chapter 5, arose in part to contest such portrayals.

Finally, as will also become clear in the chapters that follow, psychiatry and mental health are marked by what philosophers in this area describe as a pervasive problem of 'kinds.' At the risk of drastically oversimplifying a complex issue, this turns on whether psychiatric disorders are 'natural' kinds—that is, things that exist in the world independently of our description of them—or whether they are 'artificial' or 'conventional' or 'socially-constructed' kinds—categories that are formed not in spite of but due to our description of them. The implications of this question undergird the history of psychiatry as a whole, and are evidenced by shifting theories of causation and therapies, as well as the ambitious nosological projects of the nineteenth-century German psychiatrist Emil Kraepelin and the authors of the American Psychiatric Association's *Diagnostic and Statistical Manual* (DSM), among others.[42] Moreover, the pendulum swings between 'biological' worldviews on one hand and 'psychogenic' schemas on the other, so characteristic of twentieth-century psychiatry, produced an unsatisfactory binary that solidified as psychiatry became more rigorously medicalised, and that remains unresolved despite hopes that psychopharmaceuticals and then neuroimaging would furnish definitive evidence of psychiatric illnesses' biological substrate and associated causal mechanisms. Yet because knowledge about the causal mechanisms that underlie psychiatric disorders is imperfect; because there is no single procedure that will verify the existence of a mental disorder independent of a clinician's subjective judgement; and because patients' responses to treatments can vary so widely, it is still not possible to say that all psychiatric disorders are natural kinds, though some theorists argue that a strong case can be made for serious conditions like schizophrenia.[43] Instead, as the history of the DSM demonstrates, diagnoses remain essentially descriptive, and can therefore be organised and classified in various ways, independent of their (mostly inscrutable) animating mechanisms. For that reason, it is all the more important to chart the history of these developments, as they structure the key conceptions of psychiatry and mental health more broadly.

To do this, my approach is thematic but also broadly chronological. In Chapter 1, 'Walls,' I explore the rise and fall of the asylum through the prism of constant reform efforts. The waning of these institutions in the decades after the Second World War signalled the reorientation of psychiatry away from the management of the institutionalised insane, who were incorporated into a larger group of mentally ill people destined to be managed in the community. I suggest that perpetual attempts at reforming these institutions reflect the fundamental and perhaps irrevocable dilemma of how to render a carceral situation therapeutic. While in one sense the process of deinstitutionalisation can be understood as the culminating renunciation of that aim, I also argue that in the present day, prisons and aged care facilities reproduce the paradoxes and tendencies of the asylums of old.

The development of antipsychotic medications in the 1950s was an important though not uncomplicated factor in the end of the asylum. In Chapter 2, 'Cures,' I discuss the rise of these 'biological' treatments for mental illness and the broader consequences for psychiatry in the second half of the twentieth century, emphasising the shift from the somatic treatments developed in interwar European asylums to the rise of psychopharmaceuticals in the post-war decades. The parallel reorientation from outright cures to maintenance and management helped collapse the distinction between madness and other forms of mental disorder into a single category of 'mental illness' that was increasingly glossed as the equivalent of a biological disease state. The resulting biomedicalisation of psychiatry and adjacent disciplines challenged the credibility of psychoanalysis as a scientific endeavour, prompting a seismic change in official diagnostic categories while also elevating modified, standardised psychotherapies like cognitive behavioural therapy (CBT) as alternatives to classical psychoanalysis. These changes also centred the brain, rather than the mind, as the seat of mental distress and indeed, beginning in the 1990s, advances in neuroimaging seemed to promise greater insight into the mysteries of this organ. Yet as I discuss in the final section of the chapter, the most recent developments in neuroscience indicate that the brain might best be understood as a 'biocultural' entity, a conceit that also offers more nuance to strictly biomedical frameworks.

Chapters 3 and 4 move away from strictly clinical spaces to consider the direct links between psychiatry, mental health, the nation state, and international governance. Chapter 3, 'States,' outlines nations' growing interests in mental hygiene and mental health from the interwar period onwards, as part of a broader interest in population health and its political implications. It places particular importance on the role of the world wars in making psychiatry useful to militaries and governments, and on the Vietnam War as the catalyst for the advent of the post-traumatic stress disorder (PTSD) diagnosis. I also use the controversies over the ethics of military psychiatry in the Vietnam War to discuss the position of psychiatry in repressive states across the twentieth century. Chapter 4, 'Universals,' continues the focus on the nation state through the history of attempts to globalise psychiatry and mental health, culminating in the contemporary 'movement for global mental health' (MGMH). To do this, I track the various iterations of psychiatry in colonial settings, in particular the racialised ethnopsychiatry pursued by Western clinicians in French North Africa and British East Africa, and the pervasive tension between the universal and the particular in structuring such frameworks. I then consider the place of psychiatry and ideas about mental health in post-war international health bodies such as the World Health Organization (WHO) and their relationship to post-war articulations of 'world citizenship.' In the last section, I explore the relationship between psychiatry, mental health, and decolonisation, including the work of contemporary Indigenous clinicians to both reformulate Western ideas about mental wellbeing and to conceptualise the legacies of colonisation in North America and Australasia. As such, both chapters demonstrate how psychiatry and mental health can be mobilised for political ends.

The final two chapters are less concerned with such direct political uses and more with the effects of political developments on the practice of psychiatry and understandings of mental health. Chapter 5, 'Discontents,' surveys controversies within the American Psychiatric Association (APA) in the 1960s and 1970s over sexuality, gender, and race, as well as the origins of mad activism and the psychiatric survivor movement in this period. I argue that in trying to undo the influence of psychoanalysis on the DSM by insisting on the salience of sociopolitical factors, the activism of this period in fact bolstered the standing of ostensibly apolitical biomedical psychiatry. The final chapter, 'Markets,' is concerned with the relationship between psychiatry, mental health, and capitalism—specifically, the way critical interpretations of capitalism have used psychiatric concepts to both critique the effects of the marketplace on the practice of psychiatry and conceptualise capitalism as advancing a species of totalising 'psychopolitics.' Here, I discuss recent renewed interest in the notion of 'burn out,' as well as the prospectively digitised, automated, algorithmic but also marketised future of mental health care.

Several caveats are necessary. While the imprecision of psychiatric diagnoses has been a source of frustration for clinicians for centuries, terms like 'mad' and 'insane' have particularly troubling histories and connotations—stigmatising labels that have been variously critiqued, contested, discarded, and reclaimed by the activists discussed in Chapter 5. While I take these objections seriously and have put these terms in quotation marks where I deem it important to signal their contingency, I have not removed them altogether on the grounds that this would erase terminology some contemporary activists now embrace. Another problem of nomenclature relates to disciplinary boundaries, which blur around the so-called 'psy' disciplines (psychiatry, psychoanalysis, and psychology) and the various 'neuro' specialisms. While I have cleaved to these delineations when necessary—for example, when a clinician is explicitly identified as a psychiatrist, a psychologist, or a neurologist—in general I have used 'psychiatry' and 'psychiatric knowledge' to refer to a generalised state of expertise about mental disorders. The final matter is the book's Anglocentrism, a narrowness that reflects the centrality of Anglo-American states to the story of psychiatry and mental health I seek to tell. While my discussion of colonial and anti-colonial psychiatry in Chapter 4 also reflects the global influence of these nations, the chapter nevertheless points the reader to important scholarship broadening this worldview.

What can be gleaned about mental health and psychiatry in the present from scrutinising its history? While I consider this question again in the Conclusion, for now I would point to both the pervasiveness but also the ambiguity of mental health in contemporary discourse, a ubiquity that renders it a concept implicating nearly everyone. Recent publications of the WHO, for example, describe mental health as existing on a 'complex continuum,' one that is 'experienced differently from one person to the next, with varying degrees of difficulty and distress and potentially very different social and clinical outcomes,' and as something more than the mere absence of mental illness, which affects one in eight people. In the WHO's Comprehensive Mental Health Action Plan, it is a 'state of wellbeing in which the individual realises his or her own abilities, can cope with the normal stresses of life, can work productively and fruitfully, and is able to make a contribution to his or her community.' In another report, it is simply described as a 'right.'[44]

Such imprecision presents a problem. In an essay published in the *New York Times* in September 2022, psychologist Huw Green recalled receiving a referral letter outlining the medical history of a patient with severe depression. According to the referring physician, this patient had 'a history of mental health'—not mental *illness*, Green emphasised, or mental health *problems*, but mental health itself. That the term is now used to denote 'both wellness and distress,' Green argued, indicates that it is a euphemism, which is 'what we use when we want to obscure something.' For Green, while the term presents as destigmatising terminology, it also functions to disguise those things about mental illness that make us most uncomfortable, including the reality of serious, chronic conditions like schizophrenia.[45] Green's essay thus articulates a dismaying possibility: that all our mental health talk—the awareness campaigns, the anti-stigma actions, the manifold wellbeing initiatives in schools and workplaces—has diverted our attention and resources from those who are the most unwell and least able to consistently advocate for themselves.[46]

Green's essay also echoed another, oft-voiced concern: that 'mental health' not only obscures the difficult reality of some of the mental illnesses it purports to enfold, but that it recategorises an ever-widening array of emotions and behaviours, such as grief or shyness, as biomedical objects—a development abetted by what a former chair of the DSM taskforce dubbed 'diagnostic exuberance.'[47] In this way, we all have a history of mental health. Of course, the charge that decadent modern societies, allergic to discomfort, have 'medicalised' ordinary emotions is not a new one.[48] Yet the COVID-19 pandemic and its still unfurling mental health effects have re-energised and reformulated this claim into a third distinct grounds of critique: that the expansion of the mental health category serves to medicalise and thereby individualise the very real distress caused by extraneous factors such as pandemics, racial violence, and other forms of social and political injustice.[49] In this telling, the seemingly inexorable rise in the number of people diagnosed with mental illnesses is not a sign of overzealous diagnosis or generational softening, but evidence that systemic dysfunctions can produce mental distress that compels political responses. Writing in the same *New York Times* essay series as Green, the anthropologist and historian Danielle Carr suggested that insofar as chronic stress appears to increase individuals' susceptibility to mental illness, addressing these rising rates in the United States requires not just increasing the availability of mental health care, but providing better access to 'housing, food security, education, child care, job security, the right to organise for more humane workplaces and substantive action on the imminent climate apocalypse.'[50] A critical history impels similar scrutiny to past intersections of mental health, psychiatry, and politics. In 1766, John Monro's first case for the year was a patient called Flora, an enslaved woman from the Caribbean, sent to Mr Miles' madhouse-feverish, but perhaps also 'frighten'd by the ill usage of some servants in the house where she had been.'[51] A critical history of mental health and psychiatry regards her enslavement and displacement as inseparable from the mental distress Monro was summoned to treat. This book proceeds on that conviction.

Notes

1 Jonathan Andrews and Andrew Scull, *Customers and Patrons of the Mad-Trade: The Management of Lunacy in Eighteenth-Century London* (University of California Press, 2003), xi–xii, and 16. On Bethlem (also Bethlehem) Hospital see the companion volume, Johnathan Andrews and Andrew Scull, *Undertaker of the Mind: John Monro and*

Mad-Doctoring in Eighteenth-Century England (University of California Press, 2001), 20–40. On 'mad-doctoring' generally see Andrew Scull, Nicholas Hervey, and Charlotte MacKenzie, *Masters of Bedlam: The Transformation of the Mad-Doctoring Trade* (Princeton University Press, 2014).
2 On the Monro dynasty see Andrews and Scull, *Undertaker of the Mind*, 4–7.
3 For a helpful overview of relevant scholarship and the importance of the long eighteenth century to the rise of the madhouse see Leonard Smith, *Private Madhouses in England, 1640–1815: Commercialised Care for the Insane* (Palgrave, 2020), 1–17. On the Duffield and Miles madhouses, which appear in the casebook, see Smith, *Private Madhouses*, 51, 54–56.
4 Andrews and Scull, *Customers and Patrons*, 25–26.
5 Andrews and Scull, *Customers and Patrons*, 45.
6 Andrews and Scull, *Customers and Patrons*, C-105.
7 Andrews and Scull, *Customers and Patrons*, C-67.
8 Andrews and Scull, *Customers and Patrons*, C-65.
9 See George Cheyne, *The English Malady (1773)* (Routledge, 1991).
10 Andrews and Scull, *Customers and Patrons*, C-8.
11 Andrews and Scull, *Customers and Patrons*, C-9 and C-10.
12 Andrews and Scull, *Customers and Patrons*, C-55.
13 Andrews and Scull, *Customers and Patrons*, C-31 and C-32.
14 Andrews and Scull, *Customers and Patrons*, C-6 and C-7.
15 Andrews and Scull, *Undertaker of the Mind*, 19; Andrews and Scull, *Customers and Patrons*, 93.
16 Andrews and Scull, *Customers and Patrons*, C-25 and C-26.
17 Andrews and Scull, *Customers and Patrons of the Mad Trade*, 95.
18 Andrews and Scull, *Customers and Patrons*, C-31.
19 Andrews and Scull, *Customers and Patrons*, C-15 to C-17; C-29 to C-3131; C-39; C-42. On lunacy see Andrews and Scull, *Customers and Patrons*, 52.
20 Andrews and Scull, *Customers and Patrons*, C42-C43.
21 Andrews and Scull, *Customers and Patrons*, 15.
22 'The National Mental Health and the War', *Journal of Mental Science* 48, no. 200 (January 1902): 73–74.
23 'Editorial: Mental Health of School Children', *Journal of the American Medical Association* [hereafter *JAMA*], XLVII, 1, 39–40 (7 July 1906): 39.
24 Clifford Beers, *A Mind That Found Itself* (Longmans, Green, and Co., 1908), 10.
25 Beers, *A Mind That Found Itself*, 204.
26 On William James' interest in Beers see Donald Capps, 'Mental Illness, Religion, and the Rational Mind: The Case of Clifford W. Beers,' *Mental Health, Religion & Culture* 12, no. 2 (2009): 157–74; on the Phipps clinic see S.D. Lamb, *Pathologist of the Mind: Adolf Meyer and the Origins of American Psychiatry* (Johns Hopkins University Press, 2014), 99–129.
27 S.D. Lamb, *Pathologist of the Mind: Adolf Meyer and the Origins of American Psychiatry* (Johns Hopkins University Press, 2014), 88–89.
28 Gerald N. Grob, *Mental Illness and American Society, 1875–1940* (Princeton University Press, 1983), 235.
29 'The Mental Health of the School Child', *JAMA* LXIII (1914): 1225; 'Mental Health of the Child', *JAMA* 91 (4 August 1928): 345; 'Safeguarding Mental Health', *JAMA* 109, (1937): 1391; 'Mental Health: Its Principles and Practice, with Emphasis on the Treatment of Mental Deviations', *JAMA* 105, no. 7 (1935): 536.
30 'Self-Knowledge and Mental Health', *The Lancet* 212, no. 5482 (22 September 1928): 611–12; 'The Country's Mental Health', *The Lancet* 230, no. 5957 (30 October 1937): 1036–37; 'Mental Health and Disease', *British Medical Journal* 2, no. 3541 (17 November 1928): 903–04; 'Mental Health and Social Problems', *British Medical Journal* 2, no. 3592 (9 November 1929): 863–64.

31 'Mental Health in 1929: Report of the Board of Control', *The Lancet* 216, no. 5586 (20 September 1930).
32 'Foreword', *Mental Health* 1, no. 1 (January 1940): 1.
33 Laurence Brock, 'Towards a Unified Mental Health Service', *Mental Welfare* 20, no. 4 (October 1939): 93–97.
34 For an excellent discussion see Howard H. Goldman and Gerald N. Grob, 'Defining "Mental Illness" in Mental Health Policy', *Health Affairs* 25, no. 3 (2006): 737–49.
35 Marie Jahoda, *Current Concepts of Mental Health* (Basic Books, 1958), 3, 109. For a discussion of Jahoda's work as well as other attempts to define mental health see Ruth Macklin, 'Mental Health and Mental Illness: Some Problems of Definition and Conception Formation', *Philosophy of Science* (1972): 341–65.
36 On this power to detain see Tyler Durn, 'Do No Harm in Due Process—A Historical Analysis of Social Determinates of Institutionalization in the USA', *History of Psychiatry* 32, no. 4 (2021): 478–87 and also Diana Rose and Nikolas Rose, 'Is "Another" Psychiatry Possible?', *Psychological Medicine* 53, no. 1 (2023): 49.
37 For the history of psychiatry beyond the asylum see Greg Eghigian, 'Deinstitutionalizing the History of Contemporary Psychiatry', *History of Psychiatry* 22, no. 2 (2011): 201–14, and (in the same issue) Volker Hess and Benoît Majerus, 'Writing the History of Psychiatry in the 20th Century', *History of Psychiatry* 22, no. 2 (2011): 139–45.
38 Roy Porter, 'The Patient's View: Doing Medical History from Below', *Theory and Society* 14, no. 2 (1985): 175–98.
39 See Alexandra Bacopoulos-Viau and Aude Fauvel, 'The Patient's Turn: Roy Porter and Psychiatry's Tales, Thirty Years On', *Medical History* 60, no. 1 (2016): 1–18 and Flurin Condrau, 'The Patient's view Meets the Clinical Gaze', *Social History of Medicine* 20, no. 3 (2007): 225–40.
40 Condrau, 'Patient's view', 533.
41 See, for example, Sally Swartz, 'Asylum Case Records: Fact and Fiction', *Rethinking History* 22, no. 3 (2018): 289–301.
42 For an overview of the literature on Kraepelin, see Eric J. Engstrom and Matthias M. Weber, 'Making Kraepelin History: A Great Instauration?', *History of Psychiatry* 18 (2007): 267–73.
43 The scholarship here is vast but the following offer useful guidance: Christophe Gauld, 'From Psychiatric Kinds to Harmful Symptoms', *Synthese* 200 (2022): article 440, which proposes that psychiatric conditions be viewed simply as 'sets of interconnected symptoms that are harmful to the patient'; Sander Werkhoven, 'Natural Kinds of Mental Disorder', *Synthese* 199 (2021): 10135–65, which suggests that a natural kind need not have a strictly biological cause; and Jonathan Y. Tsou, 'Natural Kinds, Psychiatric Classification and the History of the *DSM*', *History of Psychiatry* 27, no. 4 (2016): 406–24, which argues against a descriptive approach to diagnoses, on the grounds that some conditions—such as schizophrenia, bipolar, depression—*are* natural kinds. See also K.S. Kendler, P. Zachar and C. Craver, 'What Kinds of Things Are Psychiatric Disorders?', *Psychological Medicine* 41 (2011): 1143–50, who propose that psychiatric disorders be understood as 'mechanistic property clusters', in which individuals share a set of complex causal mechanisms resulting in a recognisable set of symptoms, and Ian Hacking, 'Kinds of People: Moving Targets', *Proceedings of the British Academy* 151 (2007): 285–318, for a summary of the concepts that have been so influential in the history of the human sciences.
44 WHO Fact Sheet, 'Mental Health', 17 June 2022, www.who.int/news-room/fact-sheets/detail/mental-health-strengthening-our-response; WHO, 'Comprehensive Mental Health Action Plan 2013–2030, 2021, www.who.int/publications/i/item/9789240031029; WHO, 'World Mental Health Report: Transforming Mental Health for All', 2022, www.who.int/publications/i/item/9789240049338.
45 Huw Green, 'We Have Reached Peak "Mental Health"', *New York Times*, 23 September 2022.

46 On this point see Vicky Long, *Destigmatising Mental Illness? Professional Politics and Public Education in Britain, 1870–1970* (Manchester University Press, 2014), who points to a history of focusing on 'acute and minor mental health problems' rather than 'discrimination experienced by people who suffer from severe and enduring mental distress': 8.

47 Allen Frances, *Saving Normal: An Insider's Revolt Against Out of Control Psychiatric Diagnosis, DSM-5, Big Pharma, and the Medicalization of Ordinary Life* (William Morrow, 2013), 2.

48 In the 1960s and 1970s, conservative commentators like Philip Rieff and Christopher Lasch made similar charges: Philip Rieff, *The Triumph of the Therapeutic: Uses of Faith After Freud* (Penguin, 1973); Christopher Lasch, *The Culture of Narcissism: American Life in an Age of Diminishing Expectations* (Abacus, 1980). See discussion in Ian Dowbiggin, *The Quest for Mental Health: A Tale of Science, Medicine, Scandal, Sorrow, and Mass Survival* (Cambridge University Press, 2011), 157–58.

49 The pandemic's impact on mental health appears to be substantial, at least by accepted measures. The WHO's 2020 Global Burden of Disease study, for example, estimated a 27.6 per cent increase in cases of major depressive disorder and a 25.6 per cent increase in cases of anxiety disorder worldwide: see WHO, 'Scientific Brief: Mental Health and COVID-19: Early Evidence of the Pandemic's Impact', 2 March 2022, www.who.int/publications/i/item/WHO-2019-nCoV-Sci_Brief-Mental_health-2022.1.

50 Danielle Green, 'Mental Health is Political', *New York Times*, 20 September 2022.

51 Andrews and Scull, *Customers and Patrons*, C-1 and C-2.

1

WALLS

Several decades after their controversial abolition asylums are still objects of dread. At the site of the former Beechworth Asylum in rural Victoria, Australia, tour operators guide their customers through abandoned buildings in search of paranormal activity, such as the ghosts of former inmates that would furnish evidence of a brutal past.[1] Tours like this suggest the resilience of asylums in our collective imagination, their high walls concealing a cast of raving inmates and sadistic doctors. But asylums also loom large in the history of psychiatry and broader histories of mental health, a persisting interest that has generated a vast scholarly literature, as well as significant controversy over the initial purpose of these institutions—particularly evident in the ongoing contention over the adequacy of Michel Foucault's influential theory of a *grand renfermement* ('great confinement') of the insane in early modern France.[2] Similarly, the broadly accepted chronology of the asylum—a surge of private madhouses in the eighteenth century; the proliferation of large public asylums from the middle of the nineteenth century; endemic overcrowding and 'herd care' in the first half of the twentieth century; and, in the second half of the twentieth century, the final demise of the asylum under the banner of deinstitutionalisation and the unfulfilled promise of 'community care'—also conceals disagreements and uncertainties. Decades of careful scholarship suggest that any totalising account of the asylum risks flattening and obscuring an expansive and varied history, particularly when we look beyond Anglo-European contexts. Custodial responses to madness were habitual, widespread, and manifold. The asylum builders of more recent centuries have their counterparts in the ancient world, in the Near and Far East, in the early Byzantine Empire, in the Islamic Mediterranean, and in Christian Europe.[3] And because moral, religious, and medical convictions so frequently mingled with political and economic considerations, the institutions they built could be many things: places of refuge or imprisonment; sites of care or

DOI: 10.4324/9780429351464-2

cruelty; instruments of empire or postcolonial nation-building; venues of therapy or neglect; the graveyard of professional ambition or its garden. Even the buildings themselves could take many forms, so that the walls of the asylum were as often symbolic as they were real.[4] While ostensibly places of seclusion, asylums were part of the societies around them: entangled with political authority and the law, with the social life of families and communities, with notions of work and leisure, with hierarchies of race, class, and gender, and, more elusively, with the life-worlds of 'the mad' themselves.[5] Asylums might also be research venues and laboratories, sites central to the interpretation and medicalisation of madness and the concomitant professionalisation of psychiatry and allied disciplines, a process that escalated across the nineteenth century and that drew inspiration from pioneering German examples.[6] In this way, asylums foreground and prefigure the formation of the categories of mental illness and mental health, as well as mark a border between those two states.

Rather than rehearse the standard chronology, in this chapter I characterise the history of the asylum as the history of attempts to remake these institutions. In this oscillating but also escalating story of crisis and reform, repeated attempts to reconcile the custodial and the therapeutic were undermined by intertwined problems of scale (rising patient numbers and chronic underfunding) and problems of will (the habitual disdain and nihilism surrounding madness)—a self-perpetuating dynamic, accelerated by the rise of psychopharmaceuticals as discussed in Chapter 2, that culminated in widespread institutional closures from the 1970s onwards. In what follows, I trace three themes that underlie this trajectory: the centuries-long pursuit of an ever-elusive 'therapeutic community' that would transform institutions from within; the mid-twentieth century rise of sociologically inspired 'insider-outsider' critiques that challenged not only the clinical rationale for institutions but also their moral basis; and, finally, deinstitutionalisation and its aftermaths as a particularly ambivalent form of unfinished history. In terms of understanding the contemporary position of psychiatry and the rise of 'mental health' as an encompassing if contested concept, locating the asylum as a site of perpetual but unrealisable reform underscores the difficulties of applying a single template of care to those experiencing mental distress.

In search of therapeutic communities

Its longer history notwithstanding, from the second half of the eighteenth-century asylums were the subject of increasing government oversight. The character of British legislation from the mid-eighteenth century to the mid-nineteenth century is instructive here, indicating growing concern with malfeasance in private institutions (the 1774 *Act for Regulating Private Madhouses*), the provision of publicly-funded care for the indigent (the *County Asylums Act* in 1808), and aspirations to humane treatment (the 1845 *Lunacy Act*, which established the Lunacy Commission).[7] Other reform efforts were more directly therapeutic. The prime example is 'moral treatment,' a philosophy that predated the era of legal reform but anticipated elements of its spirit. In Anglophone historiography moral treatment is most usually associated with William Tuke, the Quaker superintendent of the Retreat in York, a small but celebrated establishment set in bucolic surrounds, founded in 1792. Rather than physical punishments and restraints such as chaining and flogging, the Retreat promised 'kindness' and a program of steady habits as the path back to self-control and sanity.[8] From York, the tenets of moral treatment spread to other institutions in Britain, and to Quaker establishments in the United States. The superintendent of one such institution near Philadelphia wrote that the 'settled principle of action' at his asylum was 'full conviction of the propriety of mild, but regular treatment, of attention to the dispositions and wants of the patients, of providing suitable employment and recreations, and, above all, of cherishing every ray of returning reason.'[9] Just how free patients were to resist such overtures is uncertain—hence Foucault's scepticism regarding moral treatment, which, in a characteristically uncompromising formulation, he argued had 'substituted for the free terror of madness the stifling anguish of responsibility.'[10]

There were Continental varieties of moral treatment as well. An early example comes from Florence, where Vincenzo Chiarugi pursued humanitarian reforms, albeit with 'organicist' rather than strictly 'moral' convictions.[11] Better known are the developments in revolutionary Paris, where the physician Philippe Pinel abolished chaining at the Bicêtre and the Salpêtrière (though whether he really marched into the Bicêtre to emancipate the patients himself, in an emphatic revolutionary gesture, is unclear).[12] His protégé Jean-Étienne Esquirol would go on to promote similar reforms.[13] As with the British influence in North America, this French influence also extended beyond continental Europe. The asylum movement in Brazil, for example, used the authority of French tradition and the now-mythic figure of Pinel to embark on a program of asylum building in the second half of the nineteenth century, as part of a drive for modernisation.[14]

In the context of legal reforms, the proliferation of humanitarian ideals and the state's increased interest in population health, moral treatment offered a precedent for internal institutional change allied to therapeutic goals, but its practical effects were comparatively short-lived. By the second half of the nineteenth century, many Anglo-European asylums were once again crowded and poorly funded, as well as over-reliant on 'progressive' measures of control such as straightjackets. The parlous reputation of such institutions prompted increased official scrutiny in the late nineteenth and early twentieth centuries. In Britain, additional legislation (the 1890 *Lunacy Act*, and the 1913 *Mental Deficiency Act* that created the Board of Control) plus an influx of military patients after the First World War added to this interest.[15] Then, in the interwar period, further administrative and legal changes began to prise open closed custodial models, even if the effects were not immediately obvious. Drawing on a handful of nineteenth-century precedents in general medicine and the German university clinics established in the late nineteenth century, a small number of outpatient clinics were established in large British, American, and

European cities in the interwar period.[16] The 1930 *Mental Treatment Act* in Britain (and, later, the 1946 *National Mental Health Act* in the United States), in keeping with the precepts of the mental hygiene movement, produced a new category of 'voluntary' psychiatric patient in order to encourage people to seek psychiatric treatment early, before they were 'involuntarily' admitted for long periods with more serious illnesses—although in the short term the voluntary patient legislation actually increased the asylum population.[17] This impetus for the internal reform of institutions increased after the Second World War, fostered in part by governments' high tolerance for social spending. In Britain, mental hospitals were absorbed into the National Health Service (NHS) in 1948, but the costs of administering these institutions would soon be turned into an argument for their closure.[18]

While the moral treatment of the late eighteenth and early nineteenth centuries and the impetus for humanitarian reform that accompanied it can be understood as early attempts at creating therapeutic communities, in the twentieth century the therapeutic community as a theorised entity had its origins in the Second World War. The British Army was a major innovator, for reasons both pragmatic and high-minded. It was simply not possible, in a wartime context, to provide individual psychotherapy to every man judged to need it. (Indeed, based on the First World War experience, clinicians were under substantial pressure *not* to send patients for psychotherapy, on the grounds that it might make them worse.) Group therapy in institutional settings (sometimes also called 'milieu therapy') represented a compromise—a way of reaching a larger number of patients for the same amount of effort (or even less effort, if the manner of group therapy emphasised group autonomy and self-management). As was the case with the famous Northfield experiments, as well as in Maxwell Jones' work at Mill Hill, the entire institution was theorised as a 'therapeutic community,' a microcosm of society more broadly, in which patients were encouraged to take responsibility for the running of the institution. In the more radical version practised at Northfield, there was very little conventional oversight, which reflected the social democratic commitments of psychoanalytically inclined analysts such as Wilfred Bion, S.H. Foulkes, and Tom Main. The military soon shut this down.[19] In contrast, at Mill Hill and then Southern Hospital at Dartford, the approach was more didactic, with the daily timetable broken up by lectures, work rotations, and other programmed activities.[20] By contrast, post-war American clinicians working in the Veterans Administration appear to have come to group therapy due to budgetary constraints. Overwhelmed with 'NP' (neuropsychiatric) patients, the use of groups was one way to treat more patients as the system scaled up to meet demand. In a sense, these were the forerunners of the veteran 'rap' groups that emerged during the Vietnam War and are discussed in Chapter 5. At the same time, as with the notion of therapeutic communities in general, we must be careful not to overstate their radicalism. Places like Northfield were innovative in many respects, but they also existed to serve the state (and the military) by returning the patient as a useful citizen. Nevertheless, they provided a precedent for further reform.

Developments in other jurisdictions reinforce this point. In Australia, reformist tendencies coalesced to produce a mix of hospital-specific and system-wide initiatives, most notably in the state of Victoria.[21] When the British psychiatrist E. Cunningham Dax took over the chairmanship of the Victorian Mental Hygiene Authority in 1952, a position he would hold until 1986, many of the state's mental hospitals were in dire condition, as detailed in the damning Kennedy Report of 1950.[22] Here is Cunningham Dax's account of the conditions in one Victorian mental hospital, set out in his 1961 publication *Asylum to Community*:

> The wards were mostly very dirty. . . . Chamber pots were used nearly everywhere and frequently stored during the day in the same place as the food was prepared. The smell was abominable, because straw mattresses were fairly generally used and only periodically refilled, the filthy straw being turned on to a heap. . . . The deplorable conditions were accentuated by an overcrowding in the nature of 1,500 people, many of whom were sleeping on mattresses on the floor. . . . There were few facilities for occupation, and one was confronted by the distressing spectacle of hundreds of ill-dressed people walking up and down staring at the ground within concrete or bare earth airing courts surrounded by railings.[23]

Unsurprisingly, such institutions were desperately understaffed: in 1952, nearly half of the medical positions were vacant; there were 350 fewer nurses than the minimum requirement, and there were just eight social workers in the entire system.[24] It was difficult to imagine how patients could get well in such circumstances. Cunningham Dax's response was thoroughgoing, starting with the improvement of the neglected buildings themselves and working through to patient clothing, accommodation, and daily activities. Recalibrating the institution in these ways allowed patients to 'be recognised as individuals again,' which made 'a tremendous difference to the patients' attitude to life, and their self-respect.'[25]

But this work was not just about improving facilities and staffing. For Cunningham Dax, part of reforming the asylum was breaking down both the stigma of mental illness and the sense that psychiatric hospitals and those who inhabited them were irredeemable. Instead, Cunningham Dax regarded psychiatric hospitals as one part of a 'complete service' for people experiencing mental distress, a system that encompassed both early intervention and robust aftercare, as well as better public awareness of the mental disorders and their treatment—similar ideas to those set out in Gerald Caplan's *An Approach to Community Mental Health*, also published in 1961.[26] Under Dax's leadership, the Victorian Mental Health Department began organising a Mental Health Week, on the basis that 'the stigma of mental illness largely comes from ignorance' and that by 'transmitting information to the public many of the fears can be removed and reassurance given.'[27]

Experiments occurred in other Australian states as well. One example from New South Wales is Fraser House, a therapeutic community established in the grounds of the North Ryde Psychiatric Hospital in the northern suburbs of Sydney in 1959 and overseen by the psychiatrist Neville Yeomans, who had been inspired by the work of Maxwell Jones.[28] Using 'family/friendship group therapy as the basic weapon,' Fraser House treated voluntary patients with alcohol and drug problems, as well as what were described as 'behaviour disorders.'[29] Some patients were full-time residents, others were day patients who went home at night, or who worked during the day and attended group therapy after hours.[30] While Yeomans was undoubtedly a dominating presence, patients appear to have taken substantial responsibility for the running of the unit, giving the impression of a community that was democratic if extremely rule-bound. There was a finance committee, a social committee, a 'follow-up' committee (with a post-discharge remit), and a 'Relatives and Friends Committee.' The following is the list of duties of the ward committee, the group with the greatest responsibility for the day-to-day running of the unit:

(i) being responsible for the good order of the Unit
(ii) the welfare of patients
(iii) discipline of patients
(iv) control of leave
(v) maintenance of cleanliness
(vi) cooperation with administration and staff in regard to treatment
(vii) assistance and support to new patients
(viii) it will have power with the staff to undertake locker searches and other inspections
(ix) one of the duties of the ward committee is to see that the patients keep their own clothing clean, and where a patient is unable to do his own washing or have it done, the ward committee has the obligations to see that it is done
(x) in appropriate cases, the ward committee can, after consultation with the administration and canteen committee, withhold patients' monies as security for debt or as restitution for anything stolen
(xi) As the patients' representatives, the ward committee shall co-operate with the staff in any problem of treatment, discipline, or welfare.[31]

The ward committee also had significant disciplinary powers, including oversight of a patient's leave entitlements (though staff had ultimate veto rights).[32] Patients were to be out of bed by 7.30 am every day except Sunday. Beds were to be made to hospital standard, and wards were to be cleaned and tidied each morning. Personal appearance was also important:

> Male patients will shave daily before 8.30am. All patients will be tidy by dress by that time and failure to carry out toilet and bed procedures will result in admission to the dining room being denied at breakfast. No person will be admitted to the dining room unless he or she is properly attired and this includes the wearing of slippers or shoes.[33]

Such regulations indicate that aspirations to order were not the sole province of the moral therapists, and that therapeutic communities were also disciplinary endeavours that defended the institution.

Insiders and outsiders in the asylum

While the programs of internal reform discussed above sought to improve but also strengthen institutions, more direct scrutiny of hospital processes prompted searching questions about the purpose of such institutions, including the way they influenced the course of patients' illnesses. This emerged as a key theme of post-war sociological inquiries into psychiatric care, raising questions about whether therapeutic communities within the walls of institutions were even possible. Indeed, sociologically informed research in hospitals during the 1950s and early 1960s drew conclusions not dissimilar to those later trumpeted by the radical psychiatrists and anti-psychiatrists: that the psychiatric hospital could be a damaging place, a site of rigid hierarchies and rules, somewhere that made people sicker. In one famous study of long-stay schizophrenic patients in three British hospitals undertaken during this period, the psychiatrist J.K. Wing and the sociologist G.W. Brown concluded that 'a substantial proportion, though by no means all, of the morbidity shown by long-stay schizophrenic patients in mental hospitals is a product of their environment,' a process they termed 'institutionalism.' Perhaps as worrying, however, was the potential for hospitalisation to worsen the condition of patients with less serious illnesses—what Wing and Brown described as 'secondary impairment.' Access to purposeful activity seemed determinative: 'inactivity appears to be one of the greatest dangers for the chronic schizophrenic patient and seems to be directly responsible for a certain proportion of clinical symptomatology such as flatness of affect, poverty of speech and social withdrawal.' In this sense, they argued, 'institutionalism in mental hospitals should be regarded as no different, in principle, from the condition that develops in other institutions, although it may be seen in its most severe form in long-stay schizophrenic patients.'[34]

Whereas Wing and Brown had used conventional observational methods to draw their conclusions, other studies of ward life from this period used embedded or concealed observers to uncover the inner workings of institutions and the everyday experiences of patients. While these studies indicated the influence of participant observer methodologies, they were also useful to hospital leadership. The sociologist Ivan Belknap's damning study of the poorly funded (and pseudonymous) 'Southern State Hospital,' for example, was conducted to inform a newly established central board and included data gathered by two graduate students working covertly as attendants.[35] Similarly, research undertaken at the exclusive (and later controversial) Chestnut Lodge Sanitarium was welcomed by the hospital director as a means of improving clinical administration. In this more 'open' study, patients and staff both knew that there were researchers on the ward, and the researchers themselves—a staff psychiatrist and a sociologist—stressed the importance of this collaborative approach: 'in general the personnel wanted to know the same things the investigators wanted to know, and trusted the investigators with the task of putting the facts together,' they wrote.

> If the investigators had in fact been "using" the personnel and patients as experimental objects or as instruments, a subtle but important reserve would have grown up inevitably; we suspect it would have concealed more than would have been learned from any freedom of action we would have gained.[36]

In other studies, however, concealment was paramount. A 1952 paper in the *American Journal of Orthopsychiatry* reported on a study in which a researcher was admitted to a psychiatric hospital with the knowledge of only two senior staff members. He lived on the 'less disturbed' ward for 2 months—though because he had day release privileges, he spent several hours at home every afternoon. His cover story: that he had been 'compulsively trying to finish the writing of a scholarly book, but felt he was not getting ahead,' that he had been drinking heavily and that his wife had left him. The same researcher also spent some time posing as a staff member (an assistant in the activities program). The resulting study emphasised the role of patients—notably those from upper middle-class households, fluent in the psychoanalytic orientation of the hospital—in maintaining the equilibrium of the ward, enforcing an atmosphere which discouraged 'engaging in too much immature acting-out behaviour,' 'regressing' too egregiously or denying 'the emotional basis of their illness.'[37] Studies such as these could thus surface patient agency and influence in institutional settings, not just the role of hospital procedures and staff.

This use of concealed researchers gives some context to the work of the sociologist Erving Goffman, who spent a year at St Elizabeth's Hospital in Washington D.C. posing as an assistant to the physical education instructor before writing the enormously influential *Asylums* (1961), a book that shaped perceptions of these institutions for several decades afterwards.[38] In four long essays, Goffman proposed that asylums should be understood as 'total institutions' that prompted a patient's 'self-mortification,' that a patient's 'moral career' was characterised by betrayal and then adaptation, and that patients also participated in forms of resistance (which he termed 'secondary adjustments') that constituted the 'underlife' of such institutions. The fourth essay, however, addressed institutional psychiatrists directly, making the provocative claim that they practised not medicine so much as a 'tinkering trade' on their patient-clients. As a result, incongruity ruled:

> In many psychiatric settings, one can witness what seems to be the same central encounter between a patient and a psychiatrist: the psychiatrist begins the exchange by proffering the patient the civil regard that is owed a client, receives a response that cannot be integrated into a continuation of the conventional service interaction, and then, even while attempting to sustain some of the outward

> forms of server-client relations, must twist and squirm his way out of the predicament. All day long the psychiatric staff seems to be engaged in withdrawing from its own implicit overtures.[39]

For Goffman, then, it was not just that the asylum was objectionable as an institution but that psychiatrists themselves were incapable of initiating a genuine rapport with their patients. This heightened the moral case against such places.

In addition to the participant-observer tradition, Goffman's 'fieldwork as critique' replicated other canonical accounts of the depredations of the asylum, including those of Dorothea Dix, the journalist Albert Deutsch, and the orderlies-cum-whistle-blowers of the Civilian Public Service program who worked in American asylums during the Second World War.[40] Ken Kesey's *One Flew Over the Cuckoo's Nest* (1962) drew on his experience as an attendant in a psychiatric ward.[41] Foucault, who had trained in psychology as well as philosophy, worked in hospital settings in the 1950s before leaving, he said, 'in great personal discomfort' and resolving to write 'a history of the practices' he had witnessed.[42] And for Goffman, there was another personal connection, albeit unarticulated: his first wife, Angelica, experienced mental illness for much of their marriage, was hospitalised several times, and eventually died by suicide in 1964.[43] Personal experience thus likely informed these moral and theoretical positions, even if this was not openly communicated.

In the 1970s, the use of concealed observers took a more activist turn that reflected the influence of the anti-psychiatry movement. In one now-notorious episode, psychologist David Rosenhan claimed to have run an experiment in which eight people with no prior history of mental illness were admitted to psychiatric hospitals complaining of hearing voices saying the words 'empty,' 'hollow,' and 'thud.' According to the account given in Rosenhan's paper—memorably though not subtly titled 'On Being Sane in Insane Places'[44]—all participants were admitted as patients and spent an average of 19 days on the ward, usually with a diagnosis of schizophrenia. Apart from inventing false names and occupations, these pseudopatients were instructed to act completely normally, save for their reports of hearing voices, and cooperate with staff. Once admitted, if asked, they were to indicate that they were no longer hearing voices and that they felt better. When the pseudopatients were eventually discharged, they carried their diagnoses with them: schizophrenics in remission. 'It is clear that we cannot distinguish the sane from the insane in psychiatric hospitals,' Rosenhan thundered. 'The hospital itself imposes a special environment in which the meaning of behaviour can easily be misunderstood.'[45] While it now seems likely that Rosenhan invented his data, his account of his experiment chimed with a countercultural zeitgeist that regarded institutions (and institutional psychiatry) as oppressive and stigmatising.[46]

In Australia, by contrast, the academic psychologist Robin Winkler and his students really were conducting such clandestine research. One experiment reported in 1974 involved student volunteers gaining admission to psychiatric hospitals in

Sydney based on detailed but fictitious case histories. Winkler's approach was far more constructive than Rosenhan's, his overall tone implying that he was not looking to demolish the premise of mental illness so much as offering a new way of investigating the treatment of mental illness in public institutions, understanding the experience of mental illness itself and perhaps even designing techniques that would be part of clinical training. (This is likely why some of the more radical activists in Sydney—also seeking false admissions to psychiatric hospitals during this period—felt that Winkler was too accommodating and reformist.[47]) At the same time—and in an indication, perhaps, of where Winkler's sympathies ultimately lay—he proposed that experiments like this could also be used to inform practical resistance strategies for patients, such as 'the importance of selecting your own hospital, of not being passive in treatment, and being aware of how to be discerning about the treatment process,' as well as 'practical suggestions about alternative ways of handling oneself other than going to hospital.'[48]

Winkler also used pseudopatients to understand the provision of psychiatric care in general practice. In this scenario, two pseudopatients (one male and one female) visited 25 general practitioners to test the response of GPs to patients presenting with 'depression of psychosocial origin.' The opening sections characterised this exercise as an extension of the practice of using *simulated* patients in medical education, as pioneered by the medical educator Howard Barrows.[49] While the study was also interested in eliciting material on gender differences and GPs' political commentary in the context of imminent reforms to federal healthcare funding, the most arresting point involved the easy availability of psychotropic medication, which was prescribed in 78 per cent of visits, most often a tricyclic antidepressant and usually without warnings about drug interactions or referrals to counselling or other social services, as per the NMHRC guidelines. 'General practitioners,' the study concluded, 'are highly predisposed to prescribe in the absence of any patient request.'[50] Accordingly, '[i]t is our belief that a permanent body should be established with the cooperation of medical, research and consumer organisations, to report regularly on health care service as evaluated by systematic pseudopatient observations.'[51]

Studies conducted with undeclared pseudopatients unsettled many in the medical profession. Part of this may have been disciplinary, insofar as Rosenhan and Winkler were both psychologists criticising psychiatry, but the outrage was likely heightened by proximate controversies (in Australia, the introduction of Medibank and its impact on general practice; in the United States, the ongoing controversies in the American Psychiatric Association discussed in Chapter 5).[52] But the inversion of traditional power relations performed by lay personnel on clinicians—and, in the case of Winkler, with appeals to scientific rigour—must have been equally galling. Winkler was insistent on this point, arguing that 'double-blind drug trials and placebo controls in psychotherapy research' were justified by the fact that 'important research data can sometimes be obtained only by withholding information from subjects, as long as subjects are not harmed by this withheld information.'

Accordingly, '[t]his principle, used for research with patients as subjects, can also be used when professionals are the subject of research.'[53] Regardless, the Dean of the Faculty of Medicine at the University of New South Wales, Winkler's home institution, wrote to the *Medical Journal of Australia* to confirm that the Faculty 'was not in any way associated with this exercise' and that '[a]ll of my senior colleagues with whom I have discussed this project deprecate its nature, as reported, as much as I do.'[54] Responses to Rosenhan were similarly if not more vehement and matched his own combative tone. An editorial in the *British Medical Journal* argued that pseudopatients 'divert resources from those in need; the good will of nurses and others is abused; there is a sowing of distrust, and a new and unwelcome element is added to differential diagnosis.' Indeed, despite the difficulties in evaluating standards of care in institutions, the 'false' nature of the relationship between doctor and (pseudo)patient and the 'biased' mindset of any pseudopatient rendered any conclusions worthless.[55] Howard Barrows also felt compelled to reinforce in writing the difference between the use of simulated 'non-patients' in medical education as opposed to 'untrained patient impostors.'[56]

Yet other clinicians defended Rosenhan's investigations. One correspondent to the *Medical Journal of Australia* suggested that the denunciation of Rosenhan 'betrays a very considerable editorial anxiety' about the implications of the study.[57] Writing to the *British Medical* Journal, another psychiatrist hoped that readers would not be dissuaded from consulting this 'unusual and painstaking study,' while also adding that Rosenhan's conclusions may not have been as radical as the controversy implied. 'The actual findings of the study do not particularly surprise me after 15 years' experience in psychiatry,' he wrote; if anything, Rosenhan had underplayed the essential role of the patient in psychiatric encounters and institutional dynamics. 'In my experience,' this correspondent wrote, '[patients] often know as much and sometimes more than the staff about how the mental hospital really functions.'[58] Indeed, as we have seen, prior studies had already surfaced some of the themes Rosenhan now presented as novel: the difficulty of shaking diagnostic labels bestowed upon admission, the texture of daily life on the wards, the nature of the interactions between patients and staff, and the role of medication. Moreover, voices in the profession had always acknowledged that diagnosis and treatment of patients were often more art than science; in that respect, as one recent commentator has astutely observed, Rosenhan was 'like a lawyer framing a guilty man'—an observation that is doubly resonant now it is apparent that Rosenhan fabricated his study[59]

A final observation goes to the ultimate aims of the pseudopatient studies. What Rosenhan was really investigating was not the (reasonable if unanswerable) question, he posed at the beginning of his article, a question that was also a problem of kinds—'If sanity and insanity exist, how shall we know them?'. Rather, it was something slightly different: whether psychiatrists could distinguish lying patients from truthful ones. Winkler's study of general practitioners, too, stemmed from this unspoken assumption: that doctors ought to be able to detect ill people from 'normal' people pretending to be ill. But given that both sets of pseudopatients had presented to clinicians complaining of symptoms (hearing voices and feeling depressed), would the doctors have been right to send them away? Robert Spitzer, a key combatant in the recent diagnostic battles within the American Psychiatric Association, suggested that all Rosenhan had proved was that 'pseudopatients are not detected by psychiatrists as having simulated signs of mental illness'—an 'unremarkable finding' that did not touch on the 'serious problems' of psychiatric diagnosis.[60]

From deinstitutionalisation to new asylums

Histories of internal reform efforts within asylums, as well as escalating critiques from within and without, help us contexualise the process of deinstitutionalisation, an episode in the history of the asylum approaching the controversy of Foucault's 'great confinement' thesis. Beginning in the 1950s, patient numbers in the overcrowded public asylums of the United States, Britain, and elsewhere began to decline—a complete reversal of a trend evident in the decades before the war, when asylum populations had grown precipitously.[61] The decline gathered speed over the next 20 years, so that by the mid-1970s most health authorities in the Anglo-American countries were planning for the rolling closure of large institutions and their replacement by something akin to Gerald Caplan's 'community psychiatry': a network of local clinics that would care for patients stabilised by anti-psychotic or other psychotropic medication. The scholarship points to several reasons for this change, in addition to the undeniable (but not wholesale) impact of anti-psychotic drugs, including the reorientation of the professional lives of psychiatrists towards more lucrative private practice; the increased numbers of psychologists, social workers, and occupational therapists able to help people in the community; and the fiscal (but also existential) crisis of the post-war welfare state.[62]

Some commentators have also emphasised (and indeed blamed) the influence of the anti-psychiatry movement for turning public, medical, and official opinion against asylums, with dire consequences for seriously ill patients.[63] This can be overstated. While prominent anti-psychiatrists like Thomas Szasz and R.D. Laing gained some fame (or notoriety) in the ferment of the 1960s and early 1970s, the movement itself was far from coherent.[64] A comparison of leading lights Szasz and Laing, for example, shows substantial divergence regarding the 'reality' of mental illness (Szasz denied it, whereas Laing celebrated 'madness' in certain contexts) as well as political orientation (Szasz's libertarianism against Laing's socialism).[65] These antipathies and ambivalences apply more broadly: for example, some of those dubbed anti-psychiatrists were reluctant to wear the label, preferring to call themselves 'radical' or 'critical' psychiatrists if they accepted a designation at all.[66] Finally, when considering the impact of anti-psychiatry on the fate of asylums, anti-psychiatrists' claims about these institutions were hardly unprecedented, and some of their attempts to normalise alternative communities were short-lived.[67]

Villa 21, established in 1962 at the Shenley Hospital in Hertfordshire by the radical psychiatrist David Cooper, lasted only until Cooper's resignation in 1966. R.D. Laing's community at Kingsley Hall, in London's East End, a storied establishment whose fringes melded with the arts scene and the counterculture, opened in 1965 and closed in 1970.[68] One notable exception is the revolution wrought by the psychiatrist Franco Basaglia and his colleagues in Italy in the 1960s and 1970s. Basaglia initiated a radical therapeutic community in an isolated asylum in Gorizia and then oversaw the closure of the large psychiatric hospital in Trieste, precursors to the final closure of Italian asylums altogether. Yet he also seems to have rejected the term 'anti-psychiatrist' in favour of 'non-psychiatrist'—a more accurate term for his project of abolition.[69]

The competing voices within the anti-psychiatry movement underscore that deinstitutionalisation also does not map neatly onto conventional political divisions. Leftist aversion towards institutions and authority could provide moral ballast to asylum closures, but so too could anti-welfarist conservatism, as demonstrated in Britain by Minister for Health Enoch Powell's famous 1961 'water tower' speech.[70] More broadly, focusing on a single cause for deinstitutionalisation is misleading, because the effects of several developments were culminative. Certainly psychopharmacology was important: once the new therapies were understood to be efficacious, the therapeutic rationale for longer stints in custodial care diminished further. But new administrative categories, facilitated in part by the UK *Mental Health Act* (1959) and in the United States by the *Community Mental Health Centers Act* (1963), also supported this: short-stay patients might become day patients or even outpatients if their condition could be managed by medication. Indeed, if the point of hospitalisation was assessment, there was no reason this could not be done in the psychiatric wards of general hospitals rather than in standalone institutions.[71]

Finally, on a conceptual level, the notion that one could both live in the community *and* be under psychiatric care was reinforced, and to some extent normalised (though not necessarily depathologised), by the widespread influence of psychoanalysis and other forms of psychodynamic psychology in the first half of the twentieth century. If psychopathologies were as commonplace as the psychoanalysts claimed, then the terrain between sanity and insanity was not a gaping chasm but a continuous plain, in which everything could be described as mental illness—or, indeed, as mental health. As the locus of psychiatry moved away from the asylum and towards the consulting room, as psychopharmaceuticals became a standard therapeutic intervention right across the diagnostic spectrum, and as 'mental illness' supplanted 'madness' as the discipline's primary object, the asylum became less and less defensible. In this way, deinstitutionalisation is best understood as the culmination of a series of legal and regulatory procedures and processes that, beginning in the interwar period, began to prise the asylum open. These changes were complemented by the reformist sentiment that had always run alongside the development of the asylum, the advent of antipsychotics in the 1950s and a combination of radical critique and fiscal challenges in the 1960s and 1970s.

What followed deinstitutionalisation? Here is another controversy. Because the infrastructure of 'community care' that was meant to replace the asylum never truly materialised, it is apparent that for some patients, some form of 'transinstitutionalisation' occurred—that is, that their struggles outside the asylum saw them rerouted into prisons, emergency departments, psychiatric wards, boarding houses, and homeless shelters; places Goffman would understand as total institutions.[72] It is often repeated that in the United States there are 'ten times more' mentally ill people in jail than in the care of state mental hospitals, but arriving at a definitive figure is difficult.[73] A 2014 analysis of prior studies of rates of mental illness in U.S. state prisons found that the current and lifetime prevalence of psychiatric illness was higher amongst incarcerated populations, 'sometimes by large margins.' Here, however, the problems of standardising psychiatric diagnoses also assert themselves: between the compared studies, there was a 'wide variation' in the estimated prevalence, while the 'heterogeneity in samples, states, facilities, study designs, and diagnostic instruments' employed meant that 'drawing anything more than broad conclusions about the veracity of particular prevalence estimates relative to others would be inappropriate.'[74]

In the case of prisons in the United States, however, it is difficult to disentangle the effects of the closure of asylums from the implications of a shift to a more punitive criminal justice system that prefigured the advent of mass incarceration.[75] In other words, it is not sufficient to resurrect older hypotheses about the inverse relationship between the numbers of psychiatric in-patients and the numbers of the prison population—the so-called Penrose Effect.[76] Instead, the growth of the prison population itself will necessarily increase the number of people who suffer from mental illness in prisons. Indeed, there may be a paradoxical recursive effect at work where, by sheer weight of numbers, the prison has become a primary site of mental health 'care' (and sometimes-unethical psychiatric study and experimentation).[77] In addition, by their very nature, prisons produce symptoms and behaviours that in other contexts would meet diagnostic criteria for a range of disorders. A degree of mental suffering is the point, which places prison clinicians in an anomalous position.[78] The impact of solitary confinement on the mental health of prisoners, a practice that has proliferated in the United States, provides a key example—and another instance of recursion, insofar as prisoners might be put in isolation for mental health problems.[79] Nor is it simply that segregation causes or exacerbates mental distress: prisoners with pre-existing diagnoses are also more likely to end up in solitary confinement in the first place, due to 'bizarre, annoying, or dangerous behaviour' or their difficulties in 'conform(ing) to a highly regimented routine.'[80] Thus, a new question is being asked: if prison populations decrease in response to growing critiques of the policies that created mass incarceration, where will those prisoners with serious mental illness go?[81]

While prisons have been a focus of deinstitutionalisation scholarship, a compelling argument can also be made about aged care facilities reproducing patterns of the asylum. Older people with dementia and other forms of cognitive impairment were likely always part of asylum populations, which included many patients deemed 'feeble minded' or otherwise impaired.[82] As psychiatric institutions were decommissioned, these older people were transferred to nursing homes—a shift with significant fiscal incentives, insofar as nursing home care was funded by federal rather than state governments in places like Australia and the United States.[83] Yet critics charge that poorly funded aged care facilities produce their own problems, as became apparent during the COVID pandemic.[84] Judged on the basis of psychopharmaceutical prescribing patterns, rates of mental illness in aged care are significant, a situation explained not only by increased use of antipsychotics in people suffering from behavioural symptoms linked to dementia and other forms of cognitive decline but also by a higher consumption of antidepressants and related medications by aged care residents.[85] Indeed, rates of depression in aged care facilities appear to be substantially higher compared to older people living in the community. Research on effective treatments for mental illness in the elderly also lags behind other groups.[86]

While the COVID pandemic focused attention on the deficits of residential aged care—including the psychosocial welfare of residents who were also in a kind of solitary confinement—concerns about the widespread use of psychotropic medication in these facilities have been voiced for some time. The more strident critics have accused aged care providers of practising the kinds of chemical restraint once seen in overcrowded and understaffed public asylums, and pharmaceutical companies of unscrupulous attempts to capture new markets among the elderly.[87] The prolonged use of antipsychotics for patients with dementia has come under particular scrutiny, especially the incidence of *pro re nata* or 'as-required' prescribing. Official recommendations are for short courses of treatment of up to 12 weeks once other measures have been exhausted, and the close monitoring of side effects and interactions with other medications. Yet several studies have shown that many nursing home residents are being given prolonged courses of antipsychotics due to workforce and other resourcing issues.[88]

Reform in this area is fitful, demonstrating the difficulties in governing psychiatric care across jurisdictions and specialities. In Australia, the Royal Commission into Aged Care, which predates the pandemic and was called in response to a string of public scandals about the mistreatment of aged care residents in both the private and public sectors, recommended in its final report tighter controls on the prescribing of antipsychotic medication, with the initial prescription to be written by a psychiatrist or geriatrician and then renewed by a general practitioner for up to a year.[89] However, the Australian Medical Association (AMA) successfully lobbied the Pharmaceutical Benefits Advisory Committee (PBAC) to disregard this proposal, arguing that 'GPs are well qualified to prescribe these medications' and that 'it is the environment in which antipsychotics are prescribed that needs to change as opposed to the imposition of ill-considered restrictions on prescribing.'[90] In its submissions to the Royal Commission, the AMA had reported on member concerns about antipsychotics being used as a form of chemical restraint, but also noted that only a small number of psychiatrists and geriatricians regularly visit aged care facilities, and that these specialities are particularly scarce in rural and regional areas.[91] Depriving GPs of the right to prescribe antipsychotics in the first instance would disadvantage residents who genuinely required them and, according to the AMA, undermine the role of GPs in caring for their patients. Yet the AMA submission to PBAC also acknowledged that elderly people entering nursing homes with dementia were not necessarily guaranteed continuity of primary care and that this is, in itself, a risk factor for 'an increase in polypharmacy and prescribing medicines such as antipsychotics, benzodiazepines, and antidepressants.'[92] And, indeed, in the absence of mandatory staff-to-patient ratios, low pay for staff, and high staff turnover, it is little wonder that the harried workforce lacks capacity to implement the psychosocial interventions meant to be the first recourse for agitated patients. For those who know the history of the asylum, none of this is a surprise—and, for this reason, deinstitutionalisation is unfinished history.

Conclusion

One danger of ghost tours and other forms of dark tourism in abandoned asylums is that they imply a sharp contrast with our more enlightened present. If elements of the old asylums live on in prisons and aged care facilities, as well as in group homes and other forms of residential community care, what can this tell us about the nature of our collective responses to serious forms of psychiatric distress? We are yet to build a widespread, robust infrastructure to support people with serious mental illness; until we do so, they will remain vulnerable to the suffering caused by their condition as well as the poverty, loneliness, and other forms of marginalisation that this lack of support entails. As we will see in the next chapter, while developments in psychotropic medication and in particular anti-psychotic drugs have reduced the perceived need for long-term hospitalisations, they do not constitute a universal cure so much as a means of ongoing management. In that respect, many of the challenges of humanely caring for the seriously mentally ill remain and continue to trouble the practice of psychiatry and the contemporary meanings of mental health.

Notes

1 For the Beechworth Asylum ghost tours see www.asylumghosttours.com/; for some of the history of this institution see Eileen Clark, 'Lessons from the Past: Family Involvement in Patient Admission and Discharge, Beechworth Lunatic Asylum, 1900–1912', *International Journal of Mental Health Nursing* 27, no. 1 (2018): 320–28. For the broader phenomenon of 'dark tourism' in abandoned asylums see Graham Moon, Robin Kearns and Alun Joseph, *Afterlives of the Psychiatric Asylum: Recycling Concepts, Sites and Memories* (Routledge, 2015), particularly 131–56. See also Troy Rondinone, *Nightmare Factories: The Asylum in the American Imagination* (Johns Hopkins University Press, 2019).

2 The great confinement thesis is set out in Michel Foucault, *Madness and Civilization: A History of Madness in the Age of Reason* (Pantheon, 1965). For a recent overview of the extensive scholarship on the asylum, see David Wright, 'Re-placing the Lunatic Asylum in the History of Madness', *History Australia* 19, no. 1 (2022): 161–76. For national and regional studies see Gerald N. Grob, *From Asylum to Community: Mental Health Policy in Modern America* (Princeton University Press, 1991); James Moran, *Committed to the State Asylum: Insanity and Society in Nineteenth-Century Quebec and Ontario* (McGill-Queen's University Press, 2000); Catharine Coleborne, *Madness in the Family: Insanity and Institutions in Australasian Colonial World, 1860–1914* (Routledge, 2009); and Andrew Scull, *Museums of Madness: The Social Organization of Insanity in Nineteenth-Century England* (Penguin, 1979). For an international perspective see Roy Porter and David Wright (eds.), *The Confinement of the Insane. International Perspectives, 1800–1965* (Cambridge University Press, 2003). For treatments of single institutions and individual asylum superintendents, see Anne Digby, *Madness, Morality and Medicine: A Study of the York Retreat* (Cambridge University Press, 1985) and Nancy Tomes, *A Generous Confidence: Thomas Story Kirkbride and the Art of Asylum Keeping, 1840–1883* (reprinted Cambridge University Press, 2016).

3 For an overview of approaches to madness in the ancient and medieval worlds, see Andrew Scull, *Madness in Civilisation: A Cultural History of Insanity from the Bible to Freud, from the Madhouse to Modern Medicine* (Thames and Hudson, 2015), 16–121 and 'Madness in the Ancient and Medieval Worlds' in *The Routledge History of Madness and Mental Health*, ed. Greg Eghigian (Routledge, 2017), 17–80.

4 For discussion of asylum architecture, see Carla Yanni, *The Architecture of Madness: Insane Asylums in the United States* (University of Minnesota Press, 2007) and Leslie Topp, *Freedom and the Cage: Modern Architecture and Psychiatry in Central Europe, 1890–1914* (Pennsylvania State University Press, 2017).

5 Scholarship on the social history of the asylum is extensive. For the meaning of work and importance in the institution see *Work, Psychiatry and Society, c.1750–2015*, ed. Waltraud Ernst (Manchester University Press, 2016); for the crucial role of families in mediating between patients and institutions, see Akihito Suzuki, *Madness at Home: The Psychiatrist, the Patient and the Family in England, 1820–60* (University of California Press, 2006); Coleborne, *Madness in the Family*. On the question of gender see Louise Hide, *Gender and Class in English Asylums, 1890–1914* (Palgrave Macmillan, 2014) and *Sex and Seclusion, Class and Custody: Gender and Class in the History of British and Irish Psychiatry*, ed. Jonathan Andrews and Anne Digby (Rodopi, 2004); for an analysis of race, slavery and nineteenth-century American psychiatry see Wendy Gonaver, *The Peculiar Institution and the Making of Modern Psychiatry, 1840–1880* (University of North Carolina Press, 2018); on class, see Charlotte MacKenzie, *Psychiatry for the Rich: A History of Ticehurst Private Asylum, 1792–1917* (Routledge, 1992) and *Sex and Seclusion, Class and Custody*, ed. Andrews and Digby.

6 For these research-oriented changes to nineteenth-century German psychiatry see Eric J. Engstrom, *Clinical Psychiatry in Imperial Germany: A History of Psychiatric Practice* (Cornell University Press, 2003); for a British example see Tatjana Buklijas, 'The Laboratory and the Asylum: Francis Walker Mott and the Pathological Laboratory at London County Council Lunatic Asylum, Claybury, Essex (1895–1916)', *History of Psychiatry* 28, no. 3 (2017): 311–25.

7 For an overview of this reforming era see Mark Neuendorf, *Emotions and the Making of Psychiatric Reform in Britain, c.1770–1820* (Palgrave, 2021), 1–33. For the suggestion this scrutiny constrained professionals as much as patients, see Michael Brown, 'Rethinking Early Nineteenth Century Asylum Reform', *The Historical Journal* 49, no. 2 (2006): 425–52.

8 For overviews of moral treatment see Louis Charland, 'Benevolent Theory: Moral Treatment at the York Retreat, *History of Psychiatry* 18, no. 1 (2007): 61–80; see also

Matthew McConkey, 'Human Animals: Moral Treatment and the Non-Human at York Retreat', *Literature and Medicine* 40, no. 2 (2022): 269–94.

9 Robert Waln, 'An Account of the Asylum for the Insane: Established by the Society of Friends, Near Frankford, in the Vicinity of Philadelphia', *Philadelphia Journal of the Medical and Physical Sciences* (August 1825): 15.

10 Foucault, *Madness and Civilization*, 234.

11 On Chiarugi see George Mora, 'Vincenzo Chiarugi (1759–1820) and His Psychiatric Reform in Florence in the Late 18th Century', *Journal of the History of Medicine and Allied Sciences* 14, no. 10 (1959): 424–33. For a comparison of Pinel and Chiarugi, see Donald L. Gerard, 'Chiarugi and Pinel Considered: Soul's Brain/Person's Mind', *Journal of the History of the Behavioural Sciences* 33, no. 4 (1997): 381–403.

12 For a comprehensive account of Pinel's career see Dora B. Weiner, 'Mind and Body in the Clinic: Philippe Pinel, Alexander Crichton, Dominique Esquirol, and the Birth of Psychiatry', in *The Languages of Psyche: Mind and Body in Enlightenment Thought*, ed. G.S. Rousseau (University of California Press, 1990), 331–402.

13 On Esquirol's career and legacy see Rafael Huertas, 'Between Doctrine and Clinical Practice: Nosography and Semiology in the Work of Jean-Etienne-Dominique Esquirol (1772–1840), *History of Psychiatry* 19, no. 2 (2008): 123–40.

14 Manuella Meyer, 'Sanity in the South Atlantic: The Mythos of Philippe Pinel and the Asylum Movement in Nineteenth-century Rio de Janeiro', *Atlantic Studies* 7 (2010): 473–92.

15 On the *Lunacy Act* see Akinobu Takabayashi, 'Surviving the Lunacy Act of 1890: English Psychiatrists and Professional Development during the Early Twentieth Century', *Medical History* 61, no. 2 (2017): 246–69; on the *Mental Deficiency Act* see Mathew Thomson, *The Problem of Mental Deficiency: Eugenics, Democracy, and Social Policy in Britain, c.1870–1959* (Oxford University Press, 1998), 36–76.

16 For the growth of outpatient facilities in the United States see Grob, *Mental Illness and American Society*, 238–41. For nineteenth-century precedents, see Keir Waddington, '"Unsuitable Cases": The Debate Over Outpatient Admissions, the Medical Profession and the Late-Victorian London Hospitals', *Medical History* 42 (1998): 26–46.

17 On the advent of voluntary treatment in Britain see 'Mental Treatment Act, 1930: Prepared by the Board of Control', *British Medical Journal* (10 September 1930): 139–41 and Liam Clarke, 'The Opening of Doors in British Mental Hospitals in the 1950s,' *History of Psychiatry* 4, no. 16 (1993): 527–51. For the effects of the *National Mental Health Act* in the United States see Grob, *From Asylum to Community*, 44–69. For Australia, where voluntary treatment commenced without legal change, see Milton Lewis, *Managing Madness: Psychiatry and Society in Australia 1788–1980* (AGPS Press, 1988), 34–38.

18 For an account of the organisation of psychiatric treatment in the NHS see John Turner, et al., 'The History of Mental Health Services in Modern England: Practitioner Memories and the Direction of Future Research', *Medical History* 59, no. 4 (2015): 599–624.

19 Tom Harrison, *Bion, Rickman, Foulkes and the Northfield Experiments: Advancing on a Different Front* (Jessica Kingsley Publishers, 2009) and Nafiska Thalassis, 'Soldiers in Psychiatric Therapy: The Case of Northfield Military Hospital 1942–1946', *Social History of Medicine* 20, no. 2 (2007): 351–68.

20 Maxwell Jones, 'Rehabilitation of Forces Neurosis Patients to Civilian Life', *British Medical Journal* (6 April 1946): 533–35.

21 See Lewis, *Managing Madness*, 80–81.

22 Alexander Kennedy, *Report to the Minister for Health on Mental Health and Mental Hygiene Services in the State of Victoria* (Government Printer, 1950); see also, on the role of voluntary groups, Belinda Robson, '"He Made Us Feel Special": Eric Cunningham Dax, Edith Pardy and the Reform of Mental Health Services in Victoria, 1950s and 1960s', *Australian Historical Studies* 122 (2003): 270–89.

23 E. Cunningham Dax, *Asylum to Community: The Development of the Mental Hygiene Service in Victoria, Australia* (Melbourne: F.W. Cheshire, 1961), 20.
24 For an overview of staffing levels, see Dax, *Asylum to Community*, 29–44.
25 Dax, *Asylum to Community*, 45.
26 Gerald Caplan, *An Approach to Community Mental Health* (Grune and Stratton, 1961).
27 Dax, *Asylum to Community*, 148.
28 On the North Ryde Psychiatric Hospital see Lewis, *Managing Madness*, 83. See also the summative account in Alfred W. Clark and Neville T. Yeomans, *Fraser House: Theory, Practice, and Evaluation of a Therapeutic Community* (Springer, 1969).
29 'Treatment of Alcoholics and Drug Addicts in Fraser House Neurosis and Alcoholic Unit, North Ryde Psychiatric Centre', in Neville T. Yeomans Papers, 1960–1971, State Library of New South Wales, MLMSS. 2416/2, Papers re Fraser House, 1960–1967 (hereafter 'Yeomans Papers').
30 See 'Admitting Committee', in 'Fraser House Therapeutic Community by Patients and Staff', 23, in Yeomans Papers.
31 'Fraser House: Patients' Rules for Committees', in 'Fraser House Therapeutic Community by Patients and Staff', 2–3, in Yeomans Papers.
32 'Fraser House Unit Rules—Visiting', in Fraser House Therapeutic Community by Patients and Staff', 4, in Yeomans Papers.
33 'Fraser House Unit Rules—Visiting', in Fraser House Therapeutic Community by Patients and Staff', 5, in Yeomans Papers.
34 J.K. Wing and G.W. Brown, *Institutionalism and Schizophrenia: A Comparative Study of Three Mental Hospitals* (Cambridge University Press, 1970), 184–85.
35 Ivan Belknap, *Human Problems of a State Mental Hospital* (McGraw-Hill, 1956), 3 and 6.
36 Alfred H. Stanton and Morris S. Schwartz, *The Mental Hospital: A Study of Institutional Participation in Psychiatric Illness and Treatment* (Basic Books, 1954), 448.
37 William Caudill, et al., 'Social Structure and Interaction Processes on A Psychiatric Ward', *American Journal of Orthopsychiatry* 22 (1952): 315.
38 For a contemporary view of Goffman's impact, see John Adam, et al., 'Perspectives on Erving Goffman's "Asylums" Fifty Years On', *Medicine, Health Care, and Philosophy* 16 (2013): 605–13.
39 Erving Goffman, *Asylums: Essays on the Social Situation of Mental Patients and Other Inmates* (Anchor Books, 1961).
40 Martin Halliwell, *Therapeutic Revolutions: Medicine, Psychiatry and American Culture, 1945–1970* (Rutgers University Press, 2013), 212. On Dix, see Scull, *Madness in Civilization*, 196–98; for the journalist Albert Deutsch's exposé see Deutsch, *Shame of the States* (Harcourt, 1948); on the Second World War conscientious objectors see Steven J. Taylor, *Acts of Conscience: World War II, Mental Institutions, and Religious Objectors* (Syracuse University Press, 2009); for the account of a participant see Alex Sareyan, *The Turning Point: How Men of Conscience Brought About Major Change in the Care of America's Mentally Ill* (American Psychiatric Press, 1994).
41 Kesey had worked as an attendant at the Menlo Park Veterans' Hospital in Palo Alto; see Jennifer Lambe, 'Memory Politics: Psychiatric Critique, Cultural Protest, and *One Flew Over the Cuckoo's Nest*', *Literature and Medicine* 37, no. 2 (2019): 298–324.
42 Quoted in Peter Barham, 'Foucault and the Psychiatric Practitioner', *History of the Human Sciences* 3, no. 3 (1990): 328; for relevant biographical details see Elisabetta Basso, *Young Foucault: The Lille Manuscripts on Psychopathology, Phenomenology, and Anthropology, 1952–1955* (Columbia University Press, 2022).
43 Her death is mentioned in passing in Gregory W.H. Smith, *Erving Goffman* (Routledge, 2006), 9 and Michael Hviid Jacobsen, 'Introduction: Goffman Through the Looking Glass: From "Classical" to Contemporary Goffman', in *The Contemporary Goffman*, ed. Michael Hviid Jacobsen (Routledge, 2010), 7.

44 D.L. Rosenhan, 'On Being Sane in Insane Places', *Science* 179 (1973): 250.
45 Rosenhan, 'On Being Sane in Insane Places', 257.
46 For the serious doubts as to the veracity of the experiments, see Susannah Cahalan, *The Great Pretender: The Undercover Mission that Changed Our Understanding of Madness* (Grand Central, 2019) and Andrew Scull, 'Rosenhan Revisited: Successful Scientific Fraud', *History of Psychiatry* 34, no. 2 (2023): 180–95.
47 Paul Laffey, 'Antipsychiatry in Australia: Sources for a Social and Intellectual History', *Health and History* 5, no. 2 (2003): 26–28.
48 Robin C. Winkler, 'Research into Mental Health Practice Using Pseudopatients', *Medical Journal of Australia* 2 (14 September 1974): 399–403.
49 Howard S. Barrows, 'Simulated Patients in Medical Teaching', *Canadian Medical Association Journal* 98, no. 14 (1968): 674–76.
50 Alan Owen and Robin Winkler, 'General Practitioners and Psychosocial Problems: An Evaluation Using Pseudopatients', *Medical Journal of Australia* (hereafter *MJA*) 2 (14 September 1974): 393–98.
51 Owen and Winkler, 'General Practitioners', 398.
52 Laffey, 'Antipsychiatry in Australia', 23.
53 Owen and Winkler, 'General Practitioners', 398.
54 R.J. Walsh, 'Experimental Pseudopatients', *MJA* (8 June 1974): 944.
55 'Editorial: Pseudopatients', *British Medical Journal* (hereafter *BMJ*) (28 December 1974): 729–30.
56 H.S. Barrows, 'Pseudopatients', *BMJ* (15 March 1975): 625–26.
57 See G.B. Chesher, 'Pseudopatients and Evaluation of Medical Practice', *MJA* (26 October 1974): 643.
58 D.C. Wallbridge, 'Pseudopatients', *BMJ* (8 February 1975): 334.
59 Roderick David Buchanan, 'Review of The Great Pretender: The Undercover Mission That Changed Our Understanding of Madness', *Journal of the History of the Behavioural Sciences* 56, no. 1 (2020): 53.
60 Robert L. Spitzer, 'On Pseudoscience in Science, Logic in Remission, and Psychiatric Diagnosis: A Critique of Rosenhan's "On Being Sane in Insane Places"', *Journal of Abnormal Psychology* 84, no. 5 (1975): 442–52.
61 For an overview of the rise and fall in numbers across several jurisdictions see Despo Kritsotaki, Vicky Long and Mathew Smith, 'Introduction: Deinstitutionalisation and the Pathways of Post-War Psychiatry in the Western World', in *Deinstitutionalisation and After: Post-War Psychiatry in the Western World*, ed. Despo Kritsotaki, Vicky Long and Mathew Smith (Palgrave, 2016), 22–29.
62 For a general overview of the deinstitutionalisation scholarship see Kritsotaki, Long and Smith, 'Introduction', 1–36; for figures for the United States see Grob, *Asylum to Community*, 257–61 and 268–70; for Britain see Andrew Scull, 'UK Deinstitutionalisation: Neoliberal Values and Mental Health', in *Mind, State and Society: Social History of Psychiatry and Mental Health in Britain 1960–2010*, ed. George Ikkos and Nick Bouras (Cambridge University Press, 2021), 306–14; for Australia see Robyn Dunlop and Hans Pols, 'Deinstitutionalisation and Mental Health Activism in Australia: Emerging Voices of Individuals with Lived Experience of Severe Mental Distress, 1975–1985', *History Australia* 19, no. 1 (2022): 92–114. On the fiscal and structural incentives for states to close asylums and other cognate institutions see Andrew Scull's influential *Decarceration: Community Treatment and the Deviant—A Radical View* (Prentice-Hall, 1977).
63 This is a charge put forcefully by Edward Shorter: see his *A History of Psychiatry: From the Era of the Asylum to the Age of Prozac* (John Wiley & Sons, 1997), 277.
64 For overviews of the anti-psychiatry movement see Oisin Wall, *The British Anti-psychiatrists: From Institutional Psychiatry to the Counter-culture, 1960–1971* (Routledge, 2018); Norman Dain, 'Critics and Dissenters: Reflections on "Anti-Psychiatry" in the United States', *Journal of the History of the Behavioural Sciences* 25, no. 1 (1989):

3–25, and Catherine Fussinger, '"Therapeutic Community", Psychiatry's Reformers and Antipsychiatrists: Reconsidering Changes in the Field of Psychiatry after World War II', *History of Psychiatry* 22, no. 2 (2011): 146–63.

65 Thomas Szasz railed against the 'antipsychiatry' label until the end of this life: see Szasz, 'Debunking Antipsychiatry: Laing, Law, and Largactil', *Existential Analysis* 19, no. 2 (2008): 316–44. He also reserved special animus for Laing: 'I met Laing on several occasions and he struck me, from beginning to end, as a poseur, a phoney' (ibid., 337).

66 For an overview of the different theoretical and practical tendencies that might fall under the 'anti-psychiatry' label, see John Foot, *The Man Who Closed the Asylums: Franco Basaglia and the Revolution in Mental Health Care* (Verso, 2015), 28–52.

67 On this point as it related to British anti-psychiatrists such as Laing, see Mathew Thomson, *Psychological Subjects: Identity, Culture, and Health in Twentieth-Century Britain* (Oxford, 2006), 270–71.

68 For overviews of Villa 21 and Kingsley Hall, see Wall, *The British Anti-psychiatrists*, 60–89; Adrian Chapman, 'Dwelling in Strangeness: Accounts of the Kingsley Hall Community, London (1965–1970), Established by R. D. Laing', *Journal of Medical Humanities* 42 (2021): 471–94; and Cheryl McGeachan, '"The World Is Full of Big Bad Wolves": Investigating the Experimental Therapeutic Spaces of R.D. Laing and Aaron Esterson', *History of Psychiatry* 25, no. 3 (2014): 283–98.

69 Foot, *The Man Who Closed the Asylums*, 30–31.

70 Enoch Powell, 'Address to the National Association of Mental Health Annual Conference, 9 March 1961', www.nuffieldtrust.org.uk/sites/default/files/2019-11/nhs-history-book/58-67/powell-s-water-tower-speech.html.

71 On the development of psychiatric units within general hospitals in the United States see James Walkup, 'The Psychiatric Unit Comes to the General Hospital: A History of the Movement,' *New Directions for Mental Health Services* 73 (1997): 11–23.

72 For overviews of the community care programs meant to replace institutional arrangements see Gerald N. Grob, *From Asylum to Community*, 239–72; Ian Cummins, *Mental Health Services and Community Care: A Critical History* (Bristol University Press, 2021); and Dunlop and Pols, 'Deinstitutionalisation and Mental Health Activism', 99–100.

73 The origin of this widely reported figure is the report *More Mentally Ill Persons Are in Jails and Prisons than Hospitals: A Survey of the States* (Treatment Advocacy Center, 2010), https://sanmateo.networkofcare.org/library/final_jails_v_hospitals_study1.pdf; see also Niloofar Ramezani, 'The Relationship Between Community Public Health, Behavioral Health Service Accessibility, and Mass Incarceration', *BMC Health Services Research* 22 (2022): article 966.

74 Seth J. Prins, 'Prevalence of Mental Illnesses in U.S. State Prisons: A Systematic Review', *Psychiatric Services* 65, no. 7 (2014): 866; for comparison between the USA and India see Rachel Varadarajulu and Ananya Mahapatra, 'Prisoner Mental Health in the United States of America and India: A Dual Perspective', *World Social Psychiatry* 5, no. 1 (2023): 42–46.

75 On this point see Seth J. Prins, 'Does Transinstitutionalisation Explain the Overrepresentation of People with Serious Mental Illnesses in the Criminal Justice System?', *Community Mental Health Journal* 47, no. 6 (2011): 716–22. See also the discussion in Anne Parsons, *From Asylum to Prison: Deinstitutionalisation and the Rise of Mass Incarceration after 1945* (University of North Carolina Press, 2018), 1–19 and throughout. On mass incarceration in general see Peter K. Enns, *Incarceration Nation: How the United States Became the Most Punitive Democracy in the World* (Cambridge University Press, 2016); Elizabeth Hinton, *From the War on Poverty to the War on Crime* (Harvard University Press, 2017); and Julilly Kohler-Hausmann, *Getting Tough: Welfare and Imprisonment in 1970s America* (Princeton University Press, 2017).

76 L.S. Penrose, 'Mental Disease and Crime: Outline of a Comparative Study of European Statistics', *British Journal of Medical Psychology* 18, no. 1 (1939): 1–15; for a recent

analysis see Georgina Wild, et al., 'The Penrose Hypothesis in the Second Half of the 20th Century: Investigating the Relationship Between Psychiatric Bed Numbers and the Prison Population in England Between 1960 and 2018–2019', *British Journal of Psychiatry* 220, no. 5 (2022): 295–301.

77 For a legal overview of medical experimentation (including 'therapeutic' behaviour modification and other psychiatric interventions) see Keramet Reiter, 'Experimentation on Prisoners: Persistent Dilemmas in Rights and Regulations', *California Law Review* 97, no. 2 (2009): 501–66.

78 Jeffrey L. Metzner and Jamie Fellner, 'Solitary Confinement and Mental Illness in U.S. Prisons: A Challenge for Medical Ethics', *Journal of the American Academy of Psychiatry and the Law* 38, no. 1 (March 2010): 104–08.

79 For general discussion see Keramet Reiter, et al., 'Psychological Distress in Solitary Confinement: Symptoms, Severity, and Prevalence in the United States, 2017–2018', *American Journal of Public Health* 110, Suppl 1 (2020): S56–S62; and Brandy F. Henry, 'Disparities in Use of Disciplinary Solitary Confinement by Mental Health Diagnosis, Race, Sexual Orientation, and Sex: Results from a National Survey in the United States of America', *Criminal Behaviour & Mental Health* 32, no. 2 (2022): 114–23; Nathaniel P. Morris and Jacob M. Izenberg, 'Nowhere Else to Go—Solitary Confinement as Mental Health Care', *JAMA* 330, no. 1 (2023): 17–18.

80 Metzner and Fellner, 'Solitary Confinement and Mental Illness', 105.

81 H. Richard Lamb and Linda E. Weinberger, 'Decarceration of U.S. Jails and Prisons: Where Will Persons with Serious Mental Illness Go?', *Journal of the American Academy of Psychiatry and the Law* 42, no. 4 (2014): 489–94.

82 See discussion in David Wright, *Mental Disability in Victorian England: The Earlswood Asylum 1847–1901* (Oxford University Press, 2001), 1–10; for examples from the Australian context see Brian Draper, 'Older People in Hospitals for the Insane in New South Wales, Australia, 1849–1905', *History of Psychiatry* 32, no. 4 (2021): 436–48.

83 Dunlop and Pols, 'Deinstitutionalisation and Mental Health Activism', 97–98.

84 See for example Joseph E. Ibrahim, 'COVID-19 and Residential Aged Care in Australia', *Australian Journal of Advanced Nursing* 37, no. 3 (2020): 3, and Kathy Eagar, Anita Westera and Conrad Kobel, 'Australian Residential Aged Care Is Understaffed', *Medical Journal of Australia* 212, no. 11 (2020): 507–08.e1.

85 For a discussion of prescribing patterns see Y. Yuan, et al., 'Use of Antidepressants in U.S. Nursing Home Residents: A Systematic Review', *Innovation in Aging* 2, Suppl 1 (2018): 514; Juanita Westbury, et al., 'More Action Needed: Psychotropic Prescribing in Australian Residential Aged Care', *ANZJP* 53, no. 2 (2018): 136–47.

86 For discussion see Warren D. Taylor, 'Depression in the Elderly', *New England Journal of Medicine* 371 (2014): 1228–36.

87 See for example Human Rights Watch, '"Fading Away": How Aged Care Facilities in Australia Chemically Restrain Older People with Dementia 2019, www.hrw.org/report/2019/10/15/fading-away/how-aged-care-facilities-australia-chemically-restrain-older-people#_ftn58. This report includes not just antipsychotics but benzodiazepines, sedatives and opioids as capable of constituting chemical restraint. For a helpful discussion of chemical restraint in general, see Parker Crutchfield and Michael Redinger, 'The Conditions for Ethical Chemical Restraints', *AJOB Neuroscience* 25, no. 1 (2024): 3–16.

88 For discussion see Juanita Westbury, et al., 'More Action Needed: Psychotropic Prescribing in Australian Residential Aged Care', *Australian and New Zealand Journal of Psychiatry* 53, no. 2 (2019): 136–47 and Gerard J. Byrne, 'Prescribing Psychotropic Medications in Residential Aged Care Facilities', *Medical Journal of Australia* 212, no. 7 (2020): 304–05.

89 See 'Recommendation 65: Restricted Prescription of Antipsychotics in Residential Aged Care' in Royal Commission into Aged Care Quality and Safety, *Final Report—List of Recommendations*, March 2021, 252.

90 See 'AMA Submission to Pharmaceutical Benefits Advisory Committee—Restricted Prescription of Antipsychotics in Residential Aged Care', 20 October 2021, www.ama.com.au/articles/ama-submission-pbac-restricted-prescription-antipsychotics-residential-aged-care.
91 'AMA Submission to the Royal Commission into Aged Care Quality and Safety', www.ama.com.au/sites/default/files/documents/AMA_submission_to_the_Royal_Commission_into_Aged_Care_Quality_and_Safety_FINAL.pdf.
92 'AMA Submission to Pharmaceutical Benefits Advisory Committee'; for commentary see Jeffery C.L. Looi, et al., 'Psychiatric Care Implications of the Aged Care Royal Commission: Putting the Cart Before the Horse', *ANZJP* 56, no. 1 (2022): 11–13.

2
CURES

In early May 1947, a 27-year-old woman was admitted to a hospital in Adelaide, South Australia, for treatment of what a case report in the *Medical Journal of Australia* (*MJA*) characterised as debilitating obsessional behaviour. To her treating psychiatrist, the woman had 'complained of a progressive inability to get things done':

> She was uncertain of herself and worried over everything. Had she turned off the tap in the bathroom properly? She would go back two or three times to make certain. She took hours to write a letter. She had to read and re-read it to make sure that there were no errors; the envelope must be scrutinized many times to see that the address was correct.

Though these behaviours caused her 'great distress,' she was unable to stop them. 'Her mind was constantly obsessed with anxious thoughts—of things done, being done and to be done,' the article reported. 'She had lost all confidence and always wondered whether what she did was right or not.' Previous attempts at therapy—first psychoanalysis, and then a course of electroconvulsive therapy (ECT)—had also failed. The next step was a newer and more controversial option: a prefrontal leucotomy, also referred to as a lobotomy—a neurosurgical procedure in which the surgeon cut into the white matter of the patient's frontal lobes. According to the article in the *MJA*, the patient 'unhesitatingly' agreed to the operation, 'as she could not see how "just talking" would get her well.' For 3 days after the surgery, the patient was 'very drowsy and confused,' as well as 'incontinent for some ten days,' and lacking in initiative for the next 3 weeks. But 2 months on, the article reported triumphantly, the result was 'excellent':

> The patient is completely free from anxiety and obsessions. There is no apparent intellectual loss and no failure of initiative. She is eager to get up in the morning

DOI: 10.4324/9780429351464-3

> and wants to be occupied. She is still rather slow. She is tidy and fussy, but gets things done and has no impulse "to make sure". She is punctual. She is happy and cheerful. She has no worries.

The patient's parents were reported to be 'very agreeably surprised' by this improvement, particularly her mother, 'a very precise person, who had obviously lost patience with her daughter's indecision.'[1]

The next article offered another four histories of patients who underwent prefrontal leucotomies performed by the same neurosurgeon in Adelaide, evidence of the rising profile of this procedure at the mid-century. While these operations were also deemed successful in the short term, the final outcomes were more equivocal. A young man was relieved of his depression and anxiety but 'lost his old conscientiousness and sense of responsibility,' left two jobs abruptly, and was now reported to be 'lazy' by his mother. A nun in her forties, formerly 'an amazingly clever and successful teacher,' remained in the hospital, intellectually less 'alert' although happy enough to socialise with other patients. An unmarried woman in her thirties lost her 'acute anxiety and panic' but not her aggression towards her elderly parents and had to be readmitted. The most successful case was a woman in her late forties, 'very depressed and suicidal' due to persistent delusions, anxiety and insomnia, whose symptoms appeared to completely resolve in the wake of the operation. This was a relief to the author, who had previously found her an 'importunate patient, always demanding interviews and writing letters to me. . . . [Now] she no longer worries me'—perhaps because her attention had been directed elsewhere: the neurosurgeon who had operated on her had recently received a letter from the patient, complaining of bad dreams.[2]

The mid-century clinical literature is full of such case histories, and they can tell us much about a central but comparatively understudied aspect of the history of psychiatry and mental health, one that the outsize focus on the asylum has tended to obscure: the history of therapeutics.[3] The search for cures for mental distress proceeded both within and outside the walls of the asylum, and, as I will argue in this chapter, tracing its development demonstrates the importance of therapeutics in moving the theoretical orientation of the psy disciplines towards their contemporary biomedical framework. To do this, I focus on the shift from the heroic cures developed in asylums in the first half of the twentieth century towards the psychopharmaceutical treatments of the second half of the century. A key moment in this trajectory is the development of chlorpromazine and other antipsychotics in the late 1940s and early 1950s and their (relative) effectiveness in managing the symptoms of schizophrenia, a condition that had long confounded clinicians. By stabilising patients with this condition and thus casting it as the equivalent of a discrete disease entity, the antipsychotics appeared to validate the strand of theorising that conceived of mental illnesses as 'biological'—that is, as arising from hitherto unvisualised abnormalities in the brain or in related bodily processes. In the following decades, psychoanalysis and other psychotherapeutic practices were challenged by the reconceptualisation of mental distress as biologically determined and thus amenable to biological interventions. Consequently, as we will see, psychotherapies have had to adapt themselves to new styles of biomedical reasoning and neuroscientific paradigms. Yet simultaneously, as conceptualisations of the brain and its functions become more nuanced, explanations for the production of psychiatric distress and the mechanism of effective therapies must adapt to these emerging complexities.

There are three caveats to this account. First, the therapeutic developments I trace are Anglo-European in origin, even as they made their way to other corners of the globe via transnational networks and, in many places, the imposition of colonial medicine—a history that continues to reverberate in the present. As I discuss at greater length in Chapter 4, the fact that these treatments emerge from the biomedical epistemes of the Global North and are both imposed upon and adopted by patients and clinicians in the Global South remains a source of controversy and critique. Second, while this chapter concentrates on the rise of biological treatments to the detriment of psychoanalysis, it would be remiss not to acknowledge the immense impact of psychoanalytic thought on the understandings of mental distress and mental health in the first half of the twentieth century. Even so, while there is a substantial historical literature on Freud and his circle, as well as ample scholarly material on the intellectual underpinnings of psychoanalysis, its sweeping cultural impact and its afterlife in the Anglo-European academy, it is easy to lose sight of psychoanalysis and allied psychotherapeutic techniques as a clinical practice: that is, as a method for actively *treating* certain forms of mental distress.[4] Similarly, while the characterisation of psychoanalysis as a protracted, expensive hobby of the neurotic middle classes is not entirely unfounded, historians have shown that its reach was wider: 'talking cures' were attempted in a variety of settings, including subsidised clinics for the working classes (most prevalent during the interwar period).[5] The divergence between psychoanalysis and self-consciously biological psychiatry can also be overdone. Not only is there a strong case that Freud's thought was itself 'biological,' but not all biological psychiatrists were reflexively hostile to psychoanalysis.[6] Indeed, insofar as the history of therapeutics suggests that pragmatism often ruled the day, this is hardly surprising: many practitioners were prepared to try anything with promise. Even the enthusiastic lobotomist Walter Freeman explained the efficacy of the operation as a consequence of its 'whittling down the super-ego.'[7] In this sense, psychoanalysis was more than a simple antagonist and could play an important role in theorising therapeutic effects.

Third and finally, although this chapter largely focuses on the history of how various therapies were conceptualised and first deployed, these developments cannot be separated from the contexts from which they emerged. The foregoing case histories show the deep interconnections between therapeutic choices and personal and family histories and indicate that the adoption of certain therapies and associated measures of success and failure were often situational. For this reason, a truly encompassing history of therapeutics would include not just stories of clinicians dictating treatments to uninformed or unwilling patients, but also those of patients and their families seeking relief from the anguish of mental distress and the way these choices were informed by ideas about gender, race, class, and other markers of socio-cultural significance. Accordingly, while my focus here is on the way therapeutics helped make psychiatry and mental health biological over the course of the twentieth century, I am conscious of the social and cultural histories that interleave with this shifting orientation, as well as the often unarticulated or sublimated experiences of patients themselves—an ongoing problem of finding the 'patient's view.' After her operation, the nun and brilliant former teacher leucotomised in Adelaide rose every morning, dressed and then sat 'out on the lawn or in the day room,' apparently 'calm, unworried by past or future and grateful for the relief which she has been given.'[8] We must take her doctor's word for it.

Somatic therapies in the asylum

As with the case histories that began this chapter, accounts of psychosurgery in the clinical literature are jarring to contemporary sensibilities. How should we understand these extreme and irreversible procedures? Scholars like Jack Pressman, Mical Raz, and Joel Braslow argue that psychosurgery becomes more comprehensible once we understand the broader scientific and sociocultural contexts from which it emerged as a modern technique of 'last resort.'[9] In the 1930s, influential research into brain physiology implied that the frontal lobes governed higher order executive functions and that changes to these structures could be correlated to changes in behaviour. In the laboratory led by the Yale neurophysiologist John F. Fulton, excision experiments on the brains of primates seemed to confirm the basic premise of localisation theory: that brain anatomy was roughly correlated with brain function and that targeted surgical procedures might therefore produce specific behavioural changes. Egas Moniz, the Portuguese neurologist who began prescribing prefrontal leucotomies for psychiatric patients in the mid-1930s and who won the Nobel Prize for this work in 1949, likely drew at least some of his inspiration from these Yale experiments, which Fulton and his colleague Carlyle Jacobsen presented at the 1935 International Neurological Congress in London.[10]

Wider sociocultural changes and administrative pressures also explain psychosurgery's mid-century appeal. Moniz and other proponents of psychosurgery such as the American neurologist Walter Freeman could only hypothesise as to why these brain operations might improve patients' symptoms—that perhaps they suffered from faulty brain circuity, some fixed abnormality of neuronal communication that only surgery could disrupt.[11] Yet in the absence of other effective treatments for major psychiatric disorders, the theoretical basis for these procedures mattered less than the hope they offered—to the families of suffering patients, but also to the harried staff and administrators of overcrowded psychiatric institutions, where a significant proportion of patients languished on the chronic wards.[12] This hope overrode persisting professional scepticism, a not-insignificant mortality rate and the clear evidence of significant postoperative complications and deficits for patients who survived.[13] Hope also explains psychosurgery's popularity in the psychiatric hospitals of the American Veterans' Administration, where it was characterised as a modern, scientific treatment for hitherto incurable psychiatric conditions.[14] When the alternative was presented as prolonged, perhaps lifelong institutionalisation, concomitant changes to personality and intellectual functioning were easily rationalised. This reasoning may also account for the greater proportion of women undergoing psychosurgery in institutions with otherwise equal numbers of male and female patients, insofar as the uncomplaining resumption of domestic duties was considered a therapeutic success—as in the case history that opened this chapter.[15]

While much of the scholarship on psychosurgery focuses on the American experience, it was a transnational phenomenon, suggesting that its appeal was not only a facet of post-war American enthusiasms but also a response to a broader appetite for genuine therapeutic solutions to major psychiatric illness.[16] Understood in this way, psychosurgery was not a radical departure from past practice but, rather, the culmination of several centuries of experimentation with physical or 'somatic' treatments in institutional settings, sometimes with—but often without—convincing rationales. In the early twentieth century, however, broader changes in the medical field altered the terms of engagement, so that patients, patients' families, and clinicians themselves came to expect effective, science-based remedies. Faced with very ill patients in asylums, somatic treatments thus made a kind of intuitive sense, even if their precise mechanisms remained unclear. There was, after all, a kind of conceptual consistency: an attempt to disrupt a patient's illness via the introduction of an external agent, be that a fever, a seizure, a coma, or an electric shock.

Such measures brought some relief, some of the time. Much depended on the selection of the patient. The fever therapy pioneered in the early twentieth century by the Viennese psychiatrist Julius Wagner-Jauregg, for example, had some success on neurosyphilitic patients—probably because the fever, induced by infecting the patient with malaria, attacked the syphilis bacteria itself. It showed limited effectiveness in cases of schizophrenia alone.[17] Insulin comas, initially used by the Austrian psychiatrist Manfred Sakel to help morphine addicts over the worst of their withdrawal symptoms, had moderate effects on some schizophrenic patients, though most improvements were temporary and, as with psychosurgery, entailed considerable risk.[18] Just as fever therapy sometimes ended in a fatal bout of malaria, insulin comas required vigilant nursing to keep patients sedated without suppressing their respiration entirely; mortality rates sometimes approached five per cent.[19] These constraints contributed to the spread of so-called 'convulsive therapies,' treatments that gained in popularity in European asylums in the 1930s. Intrigued by autopsy results that suggested symptomatic epilepsy might blunt the effects of schizophrenia, the Hungarian neuropsychiatrist Ladislas Meduna began injecting schizophrenic patients with camphor and then metrazol in order to produce seizures.[20] These chemical convulsions were soon superseded by electroconvulsive therapy (ECT), in which seizures were produced by currents passed through electrodes on the patient's temples. First tested by Italian clinicians in 1938 on a patient with schizophrenia, its greatest success would be in the treatment of major refractory depression.[21] But it also stood for something beyond its immediate therapeutic effects. Dubbed 'electroshock' and able to be administered by portable machines, ECT could be cast as an emphatically modern treatment—the result of a scientific, technological approach to mental illness.[22] Sceptics, however, regarded it as a sinister development, one that induced memory loss in some patients and was ripe for abuse by practitioners, who at times did indeed regard it as a disciplinary technique.[23] The controversial restrictions on the procedure in California during the 1970s and 1980s reflected these concerns.[24] Despite strong evidence for its efficacy against intractable depression, advocates have had to work hard to reverse ECT's malign image—a situation demonstrating the salience of social and cultural factors in the history of therapeutic developments.[25]

Psychopharmacology

While somatic treatments with origins in the asylum were increasingly normalised in psychiatric practice during the middle decades of the twentieth century, their reign was usurped by a more powerful claimant to the throne: psychopharmacology. Of course, the use of 'nerve tonics' or comparable substances to quell psychiatric disturbances has a long history.[26] This continuity notwithstanding, modern psychopharmacology is distinguished by its scientific stature (as verified by new forms of standardised clinical testing), its instantiation through the techniques of mass manufacture and mass marketing, and its position as a first-line therapy. It has also changed the way psychiatric disorder is theorised, contributing enormously—although not, as outlined below, unproblematically—to the notion that psychiatric disorders are 'biological' conditions akin to disease states. From the beginning, critics and sceptics have raised important questions about inflated claims of efficacy, the financial interests of powerful pharmaceutical companies and the potential for medication to obscure the social, cultural, economic, and political factors that might compromise mental health. Yet against these critiques is the undeniable impact since the 1950s of psychotropic agents on the serious psychiatric conditions that once filled the asylums, and, since the 1980s, of the consumer appetite for newer drugs that might blunt our anxiety, depression, and other forms of suffering.

The psychopharmaceutical revolution gathered pace in the decade and a half after the Second World War. First came lithium, a substance long known for its sedative properties as well as for its propensity to produce dangerous side effects. Still, its more immediate origins as a treatment for the mania of manic depression (now called bipolar disorder) were unpropitious, typical of the experimental culture of the period. In 1949, the Australian psychiatrist John Cade published a paper in the *MJA* detailing the results of lithium therapy on ten men admitted to a repatriation hospital on the outskirts of Melbourne during episodes of mania.[27] While these initial successes were tempered by the difficulties of determining an adequate maintenance dose—Cade's first patient died from lithium saturation less than a year after the article was published, one of several lithium-related deaths in Australian asylums in the early 1950s—other researchers, notably the Danish researcher Mogens Schou, carried on the work.[28] By the 1970s, there were established protocols for monitoring lithium levels with blood tests and achieving optimal doses. This meant that patients could be managed as outpatients provided they remained medication-compliant—a particular challenge with this condition, when the early phases of mania can be experienced as euphoria.[29] Lithium's clinical success also made strictly psychogenic theories of manic depression far more difficult to maintain. This was likely gratifying to Cade, who had little time for psychodynamic theorising and always maintained that major psychiatric disorders had a physiological basis. At the end of his 1949 article, he speculated on the 'possible aetiological significance of a deficiency in the body of lithium ions in the genesis of this disorder'—an example of the deficiency hypothesis sometimes used to explain the mechanism of psychopharmaceuticals.[30] In fact, it is still unclear exactly how lithium regulates mood; its effects are likely multimodal.[31]

The post-war interest in lithium coincided with a discovery of equal importance: chlorpromazine, a drug first synthesised in France in 1951 and put into preliminary use in French hospitals the following year.[32] Originally conceived as an adjunct to anaesthesia, its capacity to relieve agitation and hallucinations in psychiatric patients prompted its rapid adoption in institutions across Europe, Britain and the Americas. Chlorpromazine was the first of a new class of drugs first known as 'major tranquilisers' but eventually dubbed 'antipsychotics'—medications that could control or at least diminish patients' delusions, hallucinations, and other symptoms of psychosis. The appetite for these substances was substantial, as we might expect: the effects of prior somatic therapies were unpredictable; psychosis had hitherto proved impervious to lithium; and psychosurgery's true therapeutic benefits for schizophrenic patients were minimal. For families and clinicians caring for such patients, there were few options other than hospitalisation if patients' behaviour became unmanageable or dangerous.

The introduction of chlorpromazine as a psychiatric therapy was therefore significant in two respects. First, it gave psychiatrists a means of actively treating a group of patients who had long been the subject of so-called 'therapeutic nihilism.' Crucially, while chlorpromazine had a tranquilising effect, it did not make patients comatose or bedbound, meaning they could still participate in daily activities. Thus, as with lithium, so long as patients complied with medication protocols and were monitored appropriately, discharge from the hospital and a life in the community became thinkable, even for patients who had spent decades confined in institutions. This is not to say that the drug worked for all patients (it didn't), that there were no significant side effects (there were) or that all patients were always monitored and supported appropriately (they weren't).[33] But chlorpromazine worked *well enough*, and clinicians were eager to prescribe it, even if they retained some inner caution. For the authors of one 1956 study, '[c]hlorpromazine has been a major force in firmly launching us into the era of psychopharmacology,' though '[w]e are still suffering . . . from all the uncertainties and hesitation of a pioneer venture.'[34] In this way, the drug was not only a major driver of deinstitutionalisation, but also reshaped clinicians' relationship to schizophrenic patients themselves.

The second consequence relates to the way schizophrenia was theorised and understood. The term has a long and complex history, and the condition itself has been the subject of multiple and often contradictory theorising. It also exhibits sustained currency in non-clinical settings—not just a 'disciplinary limit point' for psychiatry, in the words of one scholar, but 'one of the most potent and politicized topoi, or themes, in the cultural theory of the late twentieth century.'[35] As with lithium, chlorpromazine stabilised not just schizophrenic patients but the condition itself, rendering it a bounded object with characteristic symptoms, seemingly amenable to a degree of chemical control. This fixity, in turn, made epidemiological study possible, both within national populations and across international borders, as we will see in Chapter 4. And, in another parallel with lithium, this occurred despite it being unclear how chlorpromazine and other antipsychotics work.[36] Its success raised the question: if even schizophrenia could be countered with psychopharmacology, what was next?

The answer was a wash of drugs aimed at combating anxiety, depression, and other varieties of what we might call 'affective,' emotional, or nervous disorders. The psychiatrist and historian Jonathan Metzl identifies three distinct waves of these 'wonder drugs,' beginning with the tranquiliser Miltown in the 1950s, followed by the benzodiazepine Valium in the 1970s, and finally Prozac, a selective serotonin reuptake inhibitor (SSRI), in the 1990s.[37] These new drugs generated new clinical and cultural effects. Compared to the heavily sedating effects of the older barbiturates, 'minor tranquilisers' like Miltown and Valium were portrayed as less sedating and less addictive—substances that dampened symptoms but did not, in theory, inhibit normal functioning. While it is difficult to determine precise prescribing and consumption patterns, these drugs gained a significant foothold in the cultural landscape of America in the 1950s and 1960s; a chemical complement, perhaps, to what some scholars have dubbed an 'age of anxiety.' They were also marketed heavily at women.[38]

After an initial surge in popularity, authorities began to urge caution. Despite their initially favourable comparisons to the barbiturates, the minor tranquilisers turned out to induce first tolerance and then addiction, suggesting they were safe only in the short term. This fact, as well as the significant side effect profile of early antidepressants like imipramine and iproniazid, provides important context for understanding the rapturous reception of SSRIs, which first appeared on the American market in the form of fluoxetine (trade name Prozac) in 1988.[39] Prozac's image as a 'clean,' precision drug—a pill that targeted only serotonin and carried no risk of addiction—made it a maintenance drug, medication a patient could safely take for years at a stable dose without inducing dependency.[40] This characterisation intertwined with another claim, one that coalesced with efforts to destigmatise mental illness but that was also easily saleable: that depression and anxiety were caused by 'chemical imbalances' in the brain and that as correctives for that imbalance, SSRIs were the equivalent of insulin for diabetics.[41] In fact, in a familiar theme, SSRIs' precise mechanism is unclear, and controversies about SSRIs' efficacy and safety, as well as the outcomes of long term use, continue to fester in clinical circles as well as patient groups.[42] The most recent controversies over the serotonin hypothesis of depression and its implications for assessing the clinical efficacy of these drugs highlight the limits of definitive knowledge in this area.[43]

SSRIs like Prozac have also generated significant cultural disquiet despite their popularity, prompting uncomfortable questions about the outsize influence of psychopharmaceutical companies on medical practice as well as the relationship between psychopharmaceuticals and the self. As the psychiatrist Peter Kramer famously argued in the bestseller *Talking to Prozac*, it may be that SSRIs make some patients feel not just normal but 'better than well,' providing a kind of 'cosmetic pharmacology' that challenges the conventional parameters of therapeutic intervention. While Kramer was captivated by some of the patient transformations he witnessed, he was also unsettled at the possibility that by prescribing Prozac he was moulding hard-driving individuals, including newly assertive women, who would serve the interests of corporate America.[44] Of course, as other commentators have pointed out, Kramer's own ideas about gender shaped his perceptions of these therapeutic encounters.[45] Yet insofar as SSRIs remain enormously popular, and insofar as it appears that women are prescribed SSRIs at far greater rates than men, acknowledging the way gender—as well as race, class, sexuality, age, and other variables—complicates the clinical profile of psychopharmaceutical agents goes some way towards positioning them as biosocial, biocultural entities.[46] In addition, the fact that most of these prescriptions are written by general practitioners underscores the profound shift in the clinical locus of psychiatry away from madness and the asylum and towards general medicine and the far larger category of mental illness. Finally, if patients now seek out psychopharmaceuticals for enhancement—Kramer's 'cosmetic pharmacology'—how does this change the stakes of psychiatry and its purposes? Renewed interest in psychedelics for improving mental health, as well as boosting overall mood and performance, will likely make these questions all the more pressing.[47]

Standardising psychotherapies

While the efficacy of lithium and antipsychotics was demonstrated by their use on asylum populations, their legitimacy was solidified by the widespread adoption of randomised control trials (RCTs) and analogous protocols in the decades after the Second World War.[48] These procedures can be understood as one example of what the historian Theodore Porter has characterised as 'technologies of trust.'[49] As more and more medicines were mass manufactured in a form to be self-administered, the RCT and related processes were critical in establishing both efficacy and consumer safety. In the case of psychiatry, however, there were even broader implications, in addition to the complexities of quantifying treatment responses and distinguishing the placebo effect in a field reliant on self-reporting.[50]

If the effectiveness of psychopharmaceuticals could be validated via RCTs, what did this mean for the various psychotherapies, whose practitioners characteristically worked closely with individual clients, often over many years? This question proved particularly urgent for psychoanalysis, a discipline that, to use historian John Forrester's formulation, reflexively 'thought in cases' and thus struggled to adapt to the statistical regimes of Anglo-American biomedicine.[51] At the end of the Second World War, psychoanalytic psychiatrists and the body of theory known as ego psychology dominated the American Psychiatric Association and most university psychiatry departments. Proponents maintained, along with Freud, that psychoanalysis was 'scientific'—that it advanced via careful observation, thorough description and the development of hypotheses that, if not always falsifiable, was at least open to scrutiny.[52] Two decades on, however, the psychopharmaceutical revolution, the validation techniques it incorporated and the rise of clinical psychology as a distinct discipline, as well as broader impatience with psychoanalysis's more ossified doctrines (discussed in more detail in Chapter 5) had begun to shake its pedestal.[53]

Adaptations were required. While some psychoanalysts began gathering data in the hope of validating their techniques, other clinicians began developing approaches more compatible with statistical confirmation.[54] Two of these would eventually form the basis of cognitive behavioural therapy (CBT), today regarded as the 'gold standard' psychotherapeutic intervention for anxiety, low-grade depression, and other affective distress.[55] (As sceptics point out, it is also the cheapest form of therapy to subsidise, appears particularly conducive to automation, and reproduces the neoliberalist trope that individual distress is a simple problem of flawed cognition.[56]) Rational emotive behaviour therapy (REBT), sometimes shortened to rational therapy (RT), was developed by the psychologist Albert Ellis in the late 1950s. Ellis contended that therapists could teach their patients 'to organize and discipline their thinking,' a self-mastery that would not only help people live 'the most self-fulfilling, creative, and emotionally satisfying lives' but that chimed with the technocratic sensibilities of Cold War America: as one scholar has noted, '[t]he "straight" thinking promoted by RT techniques' required the patient to internalise 'operationist assumptions about the primary of externalised, expert evidence over other forms of self-knowledge.'[57] Similarly, cognitive therapy (CT), developed in the early 1960s by the psychiatrist Aaron T. Beck, also promoted 'rational thinking' as the path out of mental distress; according to Beck, any intervention that altered 'faulty patterns of thinking' would qualify.[58]

While it is tempting to attribute the swift rise of RT and CT to their divergence from classical psychoanalysis and their adoption of semi-behaviourist techniques, the fracture was not absolute. Both Ellis and Beck had undertaken formal psychoanalytic training, and though Ellis soon became frustrated with what he perceived as its lack of scientific rigour, Beck saw himself as a 'neo-Freudian,' albeit one uninterested in unearthing his patients' unconscious drives.[59] Instead, what CT and RT proposed was a kind of pragmatic rapprochement between Freudian ego psychology on one hand and behaviourism on the other. Even so, there was one important difference from mid-century psychoanalysis. Like contemporary CBT, RT and CT were highly 'manualised' and thus scalable techniques: easily taught to other therapists and sufficiently standardised to be readily measurable. RT and CT were thus similar to the new psychopharmaceuticals finding their way to market in the 1960s in several crucial respects: they were compatible with RCT testing procedures, they could be self-administered, they did not require deep excavation of the meaning of symptoms and behaviours, and their focus on thinking processes anticipated the rise of both cognitive psychology and cognitive neuroscience—an observation that could also be made of contemporary neuro-inflected psychotherapies like neuro-linguistic programming (NLP) and eye movement desensitisation and reprocessing (EMDR) therapy, which both leverage their connection to the neuroscientific and situate them as biomedical interventions.[60]

Knowing the brain

While this chapter has so far sketched the ways the history of therapeutics helped make psychiatry and mental health biomedical, it is perhaps more accurate to say that both are also, now, *neuro*biological. As scholarship on the history of the neurosciences demonstrates, the advent of technologies capable of representing or visualising brain activity—electroencephalography (EEG) in the interwar period, computed topography (CT) scanning in the 1970s, and positron emission tomography (PET), magnetic resonance imaging (MRI) and finally functional magnetic resonance imaging (fMRI) from the 1990s onwards—offered researchers tantalising possibilities for understanding both the mechanisms and the manifestations of psychiatric disorder.[61] Especially after the widespread adoption of fMRI, the imminent potential to finally 'know' the brain captured both the expert and the popular imaginations, so much so that in 1990 President George Bush designated the 1990s the 'decade of the brain.'[62] Yet as a recent review of the field has emphasised, despite 30 years of hard effort, neuroimaging has 'not delivered a neurobiological account (i.e., a mechanistic explanation) for any psychiatric disorder, nor has it provided a credible imaging-based biomarker of clinical utility.'[63] One issue is scale: neuroimaging studies need large samples to be meaningful (although, as I discuss in the final chapter, new artificial intelligence capabilities might be capable of overcoming this).[64] Another is the conceptual universe in which the technologies reside. To that end, 'a full understanding of psychiatric symptoms will ultimately require integrating findings from imaging studies (which are largely correlational and anatomically coarse grained) with a rich preclinical research program that speaks to cellular and circuit-level processes.'[65]

Yet, as with the vexed questions about the mechanism of psychopharmaceuticals, this very uncertainty may yet prove generative. Rather than heralding a return to localisation theory, neuroimaging could instead support an alternative position, with important implications for the way that psychiatric disorder and mental health is represented and understood: an account of the brain as infinitely complex, inseparable from other body systems and with a propensity for constant modulation and adaption in response to endogenous and exogenous factors. Historic binaries of brain and mind, nature and nurture, and biology and culture are redundant here, because individual perceptions and experiences are vital to such a schema, as are the social and cultural circumstances in which an individual exists. Here, too, is an opportunity for transdisciplinary dialogue—and, in that spirit, I offer some possibilities from my own discipline.[66]

Historians have much to gain from thinking seriously about the brain. Certainly, the history of ideas about the brain matters very much for understanding changing notions of mental health and madness and their allied therapeutics. Spoken or unspoken, highly speculative or empirically derived, these ideas and the practices they engender can exert a powerful influence over the worldview of both patients and clinicians, as well as the institutional disposition of the therapeutic spaces in which they meet. In the past, clinicians' convictions about the brain and its capacity for both harm and healing have produced tendencies in both directions. As we have seen, the history of electroconvulsive therapy demonstrates that what is harmful in one instance (its punitive application to 'troublesome' institutionalised patients) may be lifesaving in another (its capacity to relieve intractable major depression in some individuals).[67] But ideas about the brain mattered outside clinical spaces as well. Inequalities were often naturalised via assertions about the existence of quantifiably superior and inferior brains. Imperialism, slaveholding and restricting the franchise have all been justified on such grounds, and scholarship on these topics increasingly recognises that ideas born in the clinic or laboratory can be transmitted into political discourse and popular culture in complex but highly consequential ways, often through transnational interchange.[68] Beyond the operation of overt hierarchies, ideas about the brain could be said to have exerted influence on childrearing practices, factory design, and prison reform, as well as many other social issues, particularly as psychological conceits became more explicitly biological over the course of the twentieth century.[69] In other words, to say that ideas about the brain have a history, and that that history is worth knowing, is uncontroversial. It is when we start to ask historical questions about the brain itself that thornier issues arise.

These issues were explored by historian Daniel Lord Smail in his 2008 book *On Deep History and the Brain*. In it, Smail sought not only to inaugurate a new field of 'neurohistory' but to warn historians of the perils of neglecting the implications of the 'neuroscientific and genetic revolutions of the 1990s,' thereby widening the divide between academic historians and the sensibilities of the reading public.[70] What Smail proposed was an alternative to both the reductive models of genetic destiny that dominated mainstream perceptions of neuroscience and the longstanding notion that culture is largely untethered from what we might call 'the biological.' Smail argued that historians ought to accept that there are fundamental biological parameters that broadly frame human experience and that, in particular, human brains and their associated cognitive and affective functions remain influenced by enduring biological structures and processes that have their roots in the deep 'ancestral' past. In this way, Smail's argument reflected a wider, emergent tendency amongst historians to take biology seriously: to reconceptualise the physical world and its systems as historical objects, decentre humans as the prime historical actors, and emphasise interdependence and porosity as the conditions of life.[71] As such, 'neurohistory' is an intellectual commitment as well as a methodological orientation.

Smail was careful to distance himself from the 'crude genetic determinism' characterising much of the writing on neuroscience as a means for understanding the human condition, most notably in evolutionary psychology, a discipline Smail characterises as 'naturally ahistorical.'[72] Instead, Smail suggested that what neuroscience really shows is a constant, dynamic interplay between the human 'brain–body system' and extraneous factors such as the physical environment and life experiences. This happens along two timescales. First, individual brains are modified over a lifespan, because from the moment a brain begins forming in utero it is shaped by various external contingencies that influence neural pathways (the much-discussed neuroplasticity) and gene expression (epigenetic change, which appears in some instances to be heritable, although this remains contested).[73] This process recapitulates the operation of a second, larger timescale, in which the human brain *in aggregate* is shaped by an ongoing interaction between a 'universal biological substrate' and the external world, via the process of natural selection. Importantly, the results of this interaction are not purely adaptive changes that are selected proactively. This interaction can also result in 'exaptations'—that is, changes that come to have a functional significance beyond their animating cause. Culture, for Smail, is an exaptation—and a fundamental one, insofar as it is produced by the brain but also acts upon and changes the brain.[74]

Causally speaking, then, neurohistory insists that a hard divide between biology and culture is meaningless—it is not an 'either/or,' or even a 'first this, then that,' but, rather, 'both together, all the time.' While this worldview may be universalist, it is not essentialist. If carefully deployed, it could help foster critical histories—subjecting essentialist ideas about race to profitable scrutiny, for example. In a carefully argued examination of the 'perceptual culture' of Inquisitorial Spain, Cristian Berco has posited that neurohistory can help problematise 'an inevitable cognitive link between phenotype and label' by demonstrating the role of culture in forming an individual's propensity to see in racialised types. Berco argues that because inquisitors were enjoined to assess the facial presentation of suspects, the significance of an individual's skin colour was not an automatic marker of racial difference. It thereby becomes possible to 'suggest not only that racializing categories are conceptually unstable but that they are fragile at the cognitive level.'[75]

This is not to say that there are not serious conceptual, if not moral problems that neurohistory must confront. Some of these have been carefully outlined by historians of emotions, whose own work increasingly grapples with the ontological status of their own object of study. Leading historian of the emotions William M. Reddy has very recently argued that given the number of unresolved questions about what an emotion 'is' (a sensation? an experience? prior to thought? dependent upon thought?), historians should use the term 'only provisionally,' accepting that what we call 'emotion' really refers to a 'dynamic' process in which the expression of emotion can either amplify or diminish the felt sensation.[76] In one sense, then, there is a conceptual affinity between the work of historians of emotion to historicise longstanding binaries between emotion and reason and emotion and cognition (distinctions that the neurosciences also consider simplistic), and Smail's emphasis on the 'looping' interaction between biology and culture.[77] In this regard, historian of the emotions Rob Boddice sees in the neurosciences a capacity to furnish historians, via the mechanisms of 'neuroplasticity, microevolution and epigenetics,' with 'an empirical justification for their search for experiential change over time.'[78]

Yet these affinities do not amount to an endorsement. While generally sympathetic, Boddice remains wary of what he sees as neurohistory's implicit sanction of universal, automated emotions.[79] As McGrath suggests, neurohistory's 'two-tiered historiography' can be read as trying to have it both ways: the brain is at once totally plastic and malleable but also, on another plane, fixed by its deep structures. Similarly, Reddy has argued that *Deep History and the Brain* seems 'at times bent on reintroducing functionalist explanation in a wholesale fashion,' implying that the importance Smail accords to exaptations does not displace what Reddy regards as Smail's uncritical acceptance of neuroscience as a unified and internally coherent field.[80] Likewise, Ruth Leys's penetrating attack on the state of emotions research—a field she characterises as without a clear consensus on even its 'most basic assumptions'—suggests that both Smail and Hunt risk being caught up in the overhasty rush to discard intentionality as a meaningful part of affective experience.[81] It is for this reason that McGrath argues that neurohistory is also at risk of lapsing into 'a bygone mind—body dualism.'[82]

In addition to these specific criticisms, there are two more prosaic but equally compelling concerns for historians wishing to follow Smail's lead. First, they must keep abreast of the science, an arduous task for those within the field, much less those outside it, and one complicated by fundamental and perhaps irresolvable controversies over what researchers believe we can know about the brain.[83] Second, if they are to accurately represent the state of neuroscience but argue for its usefulness nevertheless, neurohistorians must replicate something of that tentative sensibility in their own work. Reddy, in his initial review of *On Deep History and the Brain*, noted Smail's need to 'hedge' his claims to accommodate the ambiguities and uncertainties of the processes he describes.[84] Yet this may be unavoidable for authors who are rightly keen to leave the door open, intellectually speaking, to inevitable revisions of the science. Indeed, insofar as such hesitancy impedes dogma, it is probably essential for longevity. In addition, we ought to take seriously the warnings of scholars in critical neuroscience, who are rightly concerned about the overhasty instrumentalisation of tentative knowledge and its capacity to inculcate a new neuro-biopolitics.[85]

Yet here we can also heed Smail's own warnings about the propensity of neuroscience to make inflated claims that need to be scrutinised within an historicist framework. As Smail has argued, one task for neurohistorians is to speak back to neuroscientists. The point is not to argue about whether ideas about the brain have a history (an uncontroversial observation, as I have suggested, albeit one that does little to advance the empirical project in which Smail and others are engaged) but how to deal with the historicity of the brain.[86] This can be done by attending to neuroscience's 'conceptual problems' rather than its apparent solutions.[87] Pursued in this critical spirit, neurohistory need not contribute to a 'new and more insidious form of naturalization.'[88] Indeed, neurohistory may serve as an important corrective to precisely this tendency, insofar as its conceptualisation requires an acceptance of the profound and pervasive impact of culture on biology.[89]

Conclusion

In this chapter, I have proposed that changes in therapeutics over the course of the twentieth century, and particularly the advent of psychopharmaceuticals in the post-war period, produced circumstances in which mental illness was made a biomedical object: arising from the body, measurable, and capable of psychopharmaceutical management outside hospital settings. Since the 1990s, advances in the neurosciences have both reinforced this notion and complicated it. If the brain is 'embedded in interrelations between the person and the environment,' and if it is 'best seen as an organ of mediation and transformation for biological, mental, and social processes that are bound up in circular interplay,' then the claim that psychiatry is *only* 'biological' is both inaccurate and unhelpful, not just because definitive biological markers remain elusive, but because closed biological explanations cannot conceptualise the subjective experience of mental illness.[90] This more nuanced view may yet produce accounts of mental distress in which an individual's specific life circumstances and history are accorded explanatory weight equal to that of reigning disease models—a development that would hold out the possibility of more personalised, ecumenical therapies. As will become apparent in the following chapters, however, diagnostic schemas have served an important purpose in reinforcing psychiatry's prestige and require significant professional disquiet to overturn.

Notes

1 W.A. Dibden, 'Prefrontal Leucotomy for Obsessional Neurosis: Report of a Case', *Medical Journal of Australia* (25 October 1947): 511–12.

2 K.F. Edwards, 'Four Cases of Prefrontal Leucotomy', *Medical Journal of Australia* (25 October 1947): 512–16.

3 On this point see Andrew Scull, 'Somatic Treatments and the Historiography of Psychiatry', *History of Psychiatry* 5, no. 17 (1994): 1–12.
4 The scholarship on the history of psychoanalysis, its proponents and its cultural influence is voluminous. For a valuable general history see George Makari, *Revolution in Mind: The Creation of Psychoanalysis* (Duckworth Overlook, 2010); for a highly critical account see Mikkel Borch-Jacobsen and Sonu Shamdasani, *The Freud Files: An Inquiry into the History of Psychoanalysis* (Cambridge University Press, 2011); see also John Forrester, *Dispatches from the Freud Wars: Psychoanalysis and Its Passions* (Harvard University Press, 1998). For intellectual biographies of its founder, Sigmund Freud see Frank J. Sulloway, *Freud: Biologist of the Mind. Beyond the Psychiatric Legend* (Harvard University Press, 1992) and Peter Gay, *Freud: A Life for Our Time* (W.W. Norton, 2006). For the origins of its influence in American academy see Edward J.K. Gitre, 'Importing Freud: First-Wave Psychoanalysis, Interwar Social Sciences, and the Interdisciplinary Foundations of an American Social Theory', *Journal of the History of the Behavioural Sciences* 46, no. 3 (2010): 239–62.
5 See Elizabeth Danto, *Freud's Free Clinics: Psychoanalysis and Social Justice, 1918–1938* (Columbia University Press, 2005); for examples of outpatient clinics offering various forms of psychotherapies, see Suzanne Raitt, 'Early British Psychoanalysis and the Medico-Psychological Clinic', *History Workshop Journal* 58 (2004): 63–85 and Gabriel N. Mendes, *Under the Strain of Color: Harlem's Lafargue Clinic and the Promise of an Antiracist Psychiatry* (Cornell University Press, 2015).
6 Sulloway, *Freud: Biologist of the Mind*, 8.
7 Jack D. Pressman, *Last Resort: Psychosurgery and the Limits of Medicine* (Cambridge University Press, 1998), 367; see also Mical Raz, *The Lobotomy Letters: The Making of American Psychosurgery* (University of Rochester Press, 2013), 44–66.
8 Edwards, 'Four Cases of Prefrontal Leucotomy', 514.
9 See Pressman, *Last Resort*; Raz, *The Lobotomy Letters*; and Joel Braslow, *Mental Ills and Bodily Cures: Psychiatric Treatment in the First Half of the Twentieth Century* (University of California Press, 1997), particularly 125–70.
10 See Lillian B. Boettcher and Sarah T. Menacho, 'The Early Argument for Prefrontal Leucotomy: The Collision of Frontal Lobe Theory and Psychosurgery at the 1935 International Neurological Congress in London', *Neurological Focus* 43, no. 3 (2017): 1–7. On the influence of Fulton's work on the lobotomy's originators see Pressman, *Last Resort*, 47–146; on localisation theory see Katja Guenther, *Localization and Its Discontents: A Genealogy of Psychoanalysis and the Neuro Disciplines* (University of Chicago Press, 2015).
11 Raz, *The Lobotomy Letters*, 5.
12 Joel T. Braslow emphasises these factors in his work on the use of procedure in Californian state hospitals: see *Mental Ills and Bodily Cures: Psychiatric Treatment in the First Half of the Twentieth Century* (University of California Press, 1997), 125–51.
13 Incomplete records and follow-up protocols make it difficult to accurately calculate mortality rates. Work on the Umedalen Hospital in Sweden gives a mortality rate of 7.4% for operations performed between 1947 and 1960; work on the Danish figures notes rates reported in the published psychiatric literature of between 2 and 6 per cent. See Kenneth Ögren and Mikael Sandlun, 'Psychosurgery in Sweden 1944–1964', *Journal of the History of the Neurosciences* 14 (2005): 353–67; Jesper Vaczy Kragh, *Lobotomy Nation: The History of Psychosurgery and Psychiatry in Denmark* (Palgrave, 2021), 9–10. Pressman gives a mortality rate of between 1 and 3 per cent, although in light of the Scandinavian figures this may been an underestimate: *Last Resort*, 205.
14 See Pressman, *Last Resort*, 394–97.
15 Braslow, *Mental Ills and Bodily Cures*, 152–70.
16 See Brianne M. Collins and Henderikus J. Stam, 'A Transnational Perspective on Psychosurgery: Beyond Portugal and the United States', *Journal of the History of the Neurosciences* 23, no. 4 (2014): 335–54.

17 For an overview see Joel T. Braslow, 'The Influence of a Biological Therapy on Physicians' Narratives and Interrogations: The Case of General Paralysis of the Insane and Malaria Fever Therapy, 1910–1950', *Bulletin of the History of Medicine* 70, no. 4 (1996): 577–608.
18 See Robert Freudenthal and Joanna Moncrieff, '"A Landmark in Psychiatric Progress"? The Role of Evidence in the Rise and Fall of Insulin Coma Therapy', *History of Psychiatry* 33, no. 1 (2022): 65–78; for a reconstruction of workings of an insulin coma ward, see Deborah Blythe Doroshow, 'Performing a Cure for Schizophrenia: Insulin Coma Therapy on the Wards', *Journal of the History of Medicine and Allied Sciences* 62, no. 2 (2007): 213–43.
19 Freudenthal and Moncrieff, '"A Landmark in Psychiatric Progress"?', 67.
20 See Max Fink, 'Meduna and the Origins of Convulsive Therapy', *American Journal of Psychiatry* 141, no. 9 (1984): 1034–41 and Niall Mccrae, '"A Violent Thunderstorm": Cardiazol Treatment in British Mental Hospitals', *History of Psychiatry* 17 (2006): 67–90.
21 For historical overviews see also G.E. Berrios, 'The Scientific Origins of Electroconvulsive Therapy: A Conceptual History', *History of Psychiatry* viii (1997): 105–19 and Edward Shorter and David Healy, *Shock Therapy: A History of Electroconvulsive Treatment in Mental Illness* (Rutgers University Press, 2007).
22 See discussion in Laura Hirshbein and Sharmalie Sarvananda, 'History, Power, and Electricity: American Popular Magazine Accounts of Electroconvulsive Therapy, 1940–2005', *Journal of the History of the Behavioral Sciences* 44 (2008): 1–18.
23 Braslow, *Mental Ills and Bodily Cures*, 104–11.
24 For a contemporaneous discussion, see Barry Alan Kramer, 'Use of ECT in California, 1977–1983', *American Journal of Psychiatry* 142, no. 10 (1985): 1190–92. This article reflects clinician concern that patients who might have benefitted from the procedure now found it difficult to access.
25 For discussion see Jonathan Sadowsky, *Electroconvulsive Therapy in America: The Anatomy of a Medical Controversy* (Routledge, 2016).
26 See for example the chapter on nerve tonics and other treatments in Janet Oppenheim, *'Shattered Nerves': Doctors, Patients, and Depression in Victorian England* (Oxford University Press, 1991), 110–40.
27 J.F. Cade, 'Lithium Salts in the Treatment of Psychotic Excitement', *Medical Journal of Australia* 2, no. 10 (1949): 349–52.
28 See Greg De Moore and Ann Westmore, *Finding Sanity: John Cade, Lithium and the Taming of Bipolar Disorder* (Allen & Unwin, 2016); and Gordon Johnson and Sam Gershon, 'Early North American Research on Lithium', *Australian and New Zealand Journal of Psychiatry* 33 (1999): S48–S53.
29 For overviews, see Healy, *The Creation of Psychopharmacology* (Harvard University Press, 2004), 47–50 and Edward Shorter, 'The History of Lithium Therapy', *Bipolar Disorders* 11 (2009): 4–9.
30 Cade, 'Lithium Salts', 351.
31 For an overview of contemporary clinical applications see Constantin Volkmann, 'Lithium Treatment Over the Lifespan in Bipolar Disorders', *Frontiers in Psychiatry* 11 (2020): Article 377, 1–11.
32 For a comprehensive overview see David Healy, *The Creation of Psychopharmacology*, 77–101; see also Mary V. Seeman, 'History of the Dopamine Hypothesis of Antipsychotic Action', *World Journal of Psychiatry* 11, no. 7 (2021): 355–64.
33 Healy, *Creation of Psychopharmacology*, 109–10; for an early report on side-effects, including extrapyramidal symptoms, see Irvin M. Cohen, 'Complications of Chlorpromazine Therapy', *American Journal of Psychiatry* 113, no. 2 (1956): 115–21.
34 Sidney Malitz, et al., 'A Two-Year Evaluation of Chlorpromazine in Clinical Research and Practice', *American Journal of Psychiatry* 113 (1956): 544–45.
35 See Angela Woods, *The Sublime Object of Psychiatry: Schizophrenia in Clinical and Cultural Theory* (Oxford University Press, 2011), 2–3.

36 For its theorised effects on dopamine pathways, see Seeman, 'History of the Dopamine Hypothesis', 355–64 and Alan A. Baumeister, 'The Chlorpromazine Enigma', *Journal of the History of the Neurosciences* 22 (2013): 14–29.

37 Jonathan Michel Metzl, *Prozac on the Couch: Prescribing Gender in the Era of Wonder Drugs* (Duke University Press, 2003), 12–13.

38 See David Herzberg, *Happy Pills in America: From Miltown to Prozac* (Johns Hopkins University Press, 2009), 15–46 and Metzl, *Prozac on the Couch*, 127–63.

39 See the account in David Healy, *Let Them Eat Prozac: The Unhealthy Relationship Between the Pharmaceutical Industry and Depression* (New York University Press, 2004), 16–39 and Shorter, *A History of Psychiatry*, 320–24.

40 Herzberg, *Happy Pills in America*, 175–91.

41 On the evolution of the idea that depression is 'just chemical' see Jonathan Sadowsky, *The Empire of Depression: A New History* (Polity, 2021), 103–34; see also Sadowsky, 'Before and After Prozac: Psychiatry as Medicine, and the Historiography of Depression', *Culture, Medicine, and Psychiatry* 45 (2021): 479–502.

42 The psychiatrist and author David Healy has become a prominent advocate for patients reporting long-term side effects of SSRIs, including problems with sexual function. On Post-SSRI Sexual Dysfunction (PSSD) see David Healy, 'Antidepressants and Sexual Dysfunction: A History', *Journal of the Royal Society of Medicine* 113, no. 4 (2020): 133–35.

43 See Joanna Moncrieff, et al., 'The Serotonin Theory of Depression: A Systematic Umbrella Review of the Evidence', *Molecular Psychiatry* 28, no. 8 (2022): 3243–56. For a characteristic reaction and response, see Lucie Bartova, et al., 'Reply to: "The Serotonin Theory of Depression: A Systematic Umbrella Review of the Evidence", *Molecular Psychiatry* 28, no. 8 (2022): 3153–54 and Joanna Moncrieff, et al., 'The Serotonin Hypothesis of Depression: Both Long Discarded and Still Supported', *Molecular Biology* 28, no. 8 (2023): 3160–63.

44 Peter D. Kramer, *Listening to Prozac* (Fourth Estate, 1994); see also the discussion in Herzberg, *Happy Pills in America*, 175–82.

45 See for example Metzl, *Prozac on the Couch* and Judith Kegan Gardiner, 'Can Ms Prozac Talk Back? Feminism, Drugs, and Social Constructionism', *Feminist Studies* 21, no. 3 (1995): 501–17.

46 Between 2015 and 2018, around 13 per cent of Americans over the age of 18 reporting consuming anti-depressants, with higher rates for women in every age group: D.J. Brody and Q. Gu, 'Antidepressant Use Among Adults: United States, 2015–2018', *NCHS Data Brief, no 377* (National Center for Health Statistics, 2020). Prescribing patterns in England show a tripling of prescriptions for antidepressant items between 1998 and 2018, the majority for SSRIs: Paul Bogowicz, et al., 'Trends and Variation in Antidepressant Prescribing in English Primary Care: A Retrospective Longitudinal Study', *BJGP Open* 5, no. 4 (2021).

47 On the history of psychedelics see Lucas Richert, *Break on Through: Radical Psychiatry and the American Counterculture* (The MIT Press, 2019), 115–48; for some recent commentary see Collin M. Reiff, et al., 'Psychedelic-Assisted Psychotherapy', *American Journal of Psychiatry* 177 (2020): 391–420 and Alan F. Schatzberg, 'Some Comments on Psychedelic Research', *American Journal of Psychiatry* 177 (2020): 368–69.

48 For an historical overview, see Laura E. Bothwell and Scott H. Podolsky, 'The Emergence of the Randomized, Controlled Trial', *The New England Journal of Medicine* 375 (2016): 501–04.

49 Theodore Porter, *Trust in Numbers: The Pursuit of Objectivity in Science and Public Life* (Princeton University Press, 2020).

50 For a helpful overview of the complexities understanding 'improvement' in RCTs for people with non-severe depression, see Linsey McGoey, 'Profitable Failure: Antidepressant Drugs and the Triumph of Flawed Experiments', *History of the Human Sciences* 23 (2010): 58–78; see also Felix Carrier, et al., 'Ethical Challenges in Developing

Drugs for Psychiatric Disorders', *Progress in Neurobiology* 152 (2017): 58–69 and Angus Deaton and Nancy Cartwright, 'Understanding and Misunderstanding Randomised Controlled Trials', *Social Science & Medicine* 210 (2018): 2–21.

51 John Forrester, 'If p, Then What? Thinking in Cases', *History of the Human Sciences* 9, no. 3 (1996): 1–25.

52 For an overview of this perennial controversy see Agnes Petocz, 'The Scientific Status of Psychoanalysis Revisited', in *Philosophy, Science, and Psychoanalysis: A Critical Meeting*, ed. Simon Boag, Linda A.W. Brakel and Velsa Talvitie (Routledge, 2015), 145–92.

53 For the rise of clinical psychology and its relationship to broader dynamics of post-war American psychiatry see Andrew Scull, 'The Mental Health Sector and the Social Sciences in Post-World War II USA. Part 1: Total War and Its Aftermath', *History of Psychiatry* 22, no. 1 (2010): 11–14.

54 On attempts to statistically validate psychoanalytic psychotherapies see Nathan Hale, *The Rise and Crisis of Psychoanalysis in the United States: Freud and the Americans, 1917–1985* (Oxford, 1995), 300–21.

55 D. David, et al., 'Why Cognitive Behavioral Therapy Is the Current Gold Standard of Psychotherapy', *Frontiers in Psychotherapy* 9, no. 4 (2018).

56 This is put forward in Farhad Dalal, *CBT: The Cognitive Behavioural Tsunami: Managerialism, Politics and the Corruptions of Science* (Routledge, 2018).

57 Albert Ellis, 'Rational Psychotherapy', *Journal of General Psychology* 59 (1958): 35–49; see also Luke Stark, 'Albert Ellis, Rational Therapy and the Media of "Modern" Emotional Management', *History of the Human Sciences* 10 (2017): 54–74.

58 Aaron Beck, 'Cognitive Therapy: Nature and Relation to Behavior Therapy', *Behavior Therapy* 1, no. 2 (1970): 184–200.

59 Stark, 'Albert Ellis', 59; Rachael I. Rosner, 'The "Splendid Isolation" of Aaron T. Beck', *Isis* 105, no. 4 (2014): 734–58.

60 See Stark, 'Albert Ellis', 67–68; Rachel I. Rosner, 'Manualizing Psychotherapy: Aaron T. Beck and the Origins of *Cognitive Theory of Depression*', *European Journal of Psychotherapy and Counselling* 20 (2018): 25–47. On the controversial history of EMDR and its links to NLP, see Gerald M. Rosen, 'Revisiting the Origins of EMDR', *Journal of Contemporary Psychotherapy* 53 (2023): 289–96.

61 For general overviews of the efforts to visualise the brain, see Carl E. Schoonover, *Portraits of the Mind: Visualizing the Brain from Antiquity to the 21st Century* (Abrams, 2010) and Matthew Cobb, *The Idea of the Brain: A History* (Basic Books, 2021); on the development of EEG see Cornelius Bock, *Brainwaves: A Cultural History of Electroencephalography*, trans. Ann M. Hentschel (Routledge, 2018).

62 'The Decade of the Brain', *Presidential Proclamation 6158*, 17 July 1990, www.loc.gov/loc/brain/proclaim.html.

63 Matthew M. Nour, et al., 'Functional Neuroimaging in Psychiatry and the Case for Failing Better', *Neuron* 110 (2022): 2531. Most pertinently, observations do not map nicely onto diagnoses but appear common to several disorders: Zhiqiang Sha, et al., 'Common Dysfunction of Large-Scale Neurocognitive Networks Across Psychiatric Disorders', *Biological Psychiatry* 85 (2019): 379–88.

64 Scott Marek, et al., 'Reproducible Brain-wide Association Studies Require Thousands of Individuals', *Nature* 603 (2022): 654–60.

65 Nour, et al., 'Functional Neuroimaging', 2533. The kinds of questions asked about the brain are also relevant: see Joseph Dumit, 'Plastic Neuroscience: Studying What the Brain Cares About', *Frontiers in Human Neuroscience* 8 (2014): 176.

66 The following is adapted from Elizabeth Roberts-Pedersen, 'Towards a (Bio)cultural History of the Brain?', *History Australia* 19 (2022): 15–60.

67 For overviews and discussion see Simon D. Shorvon, *The Idea of Epilepsy: A Medical and Social History of Epilepsy in the Modern Era (1860–2020)* (Cambridge University Press, 2023) and Elisabeth M.S. Sherman, 'Neuropsychological Outcomes After Epilepsy Surgery: Systematic Review and Pooled Estimates', *Epilepsia* 52 (2011): 857–69.

68 Phrenology and eugenics are key examples: see James Poskett, *Materials of the Mind: Phrenology, Race, and the Global History of Science, 1815–1920* (University of Chicago Press, 2019); Marius Turda, 'New Perspectives on Race and Eugenics', *The Historical Journal* 51 (2008): 1115–24; *The Oxford Handbook of the History of Eugenics*, ed. Alison Bashford and Philippa Levine (Oxford University Press, 2010); Diane B. Paul, 'Reflections on the Historiography of American Eugenics: Trends, Fractures, Tensions', *Journal of the History of Biology* 49 (2016): 641–58.
69 See for example Marga Vicedo, *The Nature and Nurture of Love: From Imprinting to Attachment in Cold War America* (University of Chicago Press, 2013); John C. Burhman, *Accident Prone: A History of Technology, Psychology, and Misfits of the Machine Age* (University of Chicago Press, 2009); and Craig Haney, 'The Psychological Effects of Solitary Confinement: A Systematic Critique', *Crime and Justice* 47 (2018): 365–416.
70 Daniel Lord Smail, *On Deep History and the Brain* (University of California Press, 2008), 10.
71 Smail has also proposed that neurohistory can be regarded as a 'branch of environmental history': see Rob Boddice and Daniel Lord Smail, 'Neurohistory', in *Debating New Approaches to History*, ed. Marek Tamm and Peter Burke (Bloomsbury Academic, 2018), 316. For an extensive overview of some of these themes see Julie Adeney Thomas, 'History and Biology in the Anthropocene: Problems of Scale, Problems of Value', *American Historical Review* 119 (2014): 1587–607, part of the 'Roundtable: History Meets Biology' section of that issue. See also J.R. McNeil, 'Peak Document and the Future of History', *American Historical Review* 125 (2020): 1–18 for discussion of 'the mounting flood of historical evidence from the natural sciences.'
72 Smail, *On Deep History and the Brain*, 114 and 148.
73 See Max-Planck-Gesellschaft. 'Epigenetics Between the Generations: We Inherit More than Just Genes', *ScienceDaily*, www.sciencedaily.com/releases/2017/07/170717100548.htm (accessed 21 November 2021). For a general overview see S.C.P. Williams, 'Epigenetics', *PNAS* 110 (2013): 3209, although see also Mark Ptashne, 'Epigenetics: Core Misconcept', *PNAS* 110 (2013): 7101–03 and David Penny, 'Epigenetics, Darwin, and Lamarck', *Genome Biology and Evolution* 7 (2015): 1758–60.
74 Smail, *On Deep History and the Brain*, 127–30.
75 Cristian Berco, 'Perception and the Mulatto Body in Inquisitorial Spain: A Neurohistory', *Past & Present* 231 (2016): 33–60.
76 William M. Reddy, 'The Unavoidable Intentionality of Affect: The History of Emotions and the Neurosciences of the Present Day', *Emotion Review* 12 (2020): 168–78.
77 On this affinity see Larry S. McGrath, 'Historiography, Affect, and the Neurosciences', *History of Psychology* 20 (2017): 129–47. On 'looping' see Jeremy Trevelyan Burman, 'History from Within? Contextualising the New Neurohistory and Seeking Its Methods', *History of Psychology* 15 (2012): 84–99.
78 Rob Boddice, *A History of Feelings* (Reaktion, 2019), 10–11.
79 Boddice and Smail, 'Neurohistory', 307.
80 William Reddy, 'Neuroscience and the Fallacies of Functionalism', *History & Theory* 49 (2010): 413 and generally 412–25.
81 Ruth Leys, *The Ascent of Affect: Genealogy and Critique* (University of Chicago Press, 2017), 1.
82 McGrath, 'Historiography, Affect, and the Neurosciences', 142.
83 See discussion in Charles T. Wolfe, 'Introduction,' in *Brain Theory: Essays in Critical Neurophilosophy* (Palgrave, 2014), 1–13.
84 Reddy, 'Fallacies of Functionalism', 418.
85 See for example Roger Cooter, 'Neural Veils and the Will to Historical Critique: Why Historians of Science Need to Take the Neuro-Turn Seriously', *Isis* 105 (2014): 145–54; for a more measured appraisal see Nikolas Rose and Joelle M. Abi-Rached, *Neuro: The New Brain Sciences and the Management of the Mind* (Princeton University Press, 2013).

86 As Smail puts it, it is 'important for cognitive neuroscientists to learn how to come to grips with the brain's historicity': 'Neurohistory in Action: Hoarding and the Human Past', *Isis* 105 (2014): 113.
87 McGrath, 'Historiography, Affect, and the Neurosciences', 143.
88 Cooter, 'Neural Veils', 149.
89 Boddice makes a similar argument, that '[w]e can no longer think in terms of nature and nurture, but only in terms of bioculture, which is not immune to history, but mutable': Boddice and Smail, 'Neurohistory', 301–02.
90 See Thomas Fuchs, 'Are Mental Illnesses Diseases of the Brain?', in *Critical Neuroscience: A Handbook of the Social and Cultural Contexts of Neuroscience*, ed. Suparna Choudhury and Jan Slaby (Wiley, 2011), 331–44.

3

STATES

In addition to perpetual reform efforts in asylums and advances in therapeutics, the expansion of state functions impelled changes in the orientation of psychiatry and the political saliency of mental health. In particular, twentieth-century warfare accelerated the state's interest in the health of its population and the prestige and importance of medicine in general. Psychiatry and related disciplines benefitted from this tendency, particularly in Anglo-American contexts, as concern with the psychological status of fighting men increasingly embedded psychiatric knowledge into state infrastructure—not just the military and veteran entitlements, but the broader health system as well. While the effects were most pronounced after both world wars, as I will suggest below, the Vietnam War also had a significant if underappreciated impact on our psychiatric present. The special attention given to the damaged veterans of that conflict by a politicised group of clinicians, during a period in which American psychiatry was questioning its fundamental diagnostic apparatus, led to a profound shift in the way psychological trauma was understood, deployed, and legitimated by clinicians, patients, and governments in the last decades of the twentieth century. Longstanding controversies over its conceptual coherence notwithstanding, trauma and its effects now had a respectable home—in the third edition of the *Diagnostic and Statistical Manual* (DSM-III), published in 1980, as the diagnosis of 'Post Traumatic Stress Disorder' (PTSD).

The impact of mass warfare on ideas about mental health occurred in the context of growing state interest in the health of the populations they governed. Historians of public health point to two distinct if at times overlapping phases in its modern development. The first, which spans the nineteenth century and the early decades of the twentieth century, was characterised by the manipulation of the external environment to control infective agents that spread endemic illnesses like tuberculosis, smallpox, and venereal diseases. In many cases, this was effected not

DOI: 10.4324/9780429351464-4

just by sanitation works but by enforcing what the historian Alison Bashford described, in the imperial context, as 'lines of hygiene'—demarcations and containment measures like quarantine stations, fever wards, asylums, and lock hospitals that separated the healthy from the sick.[1] The second phase, which began in the early twentieth century, involved the state's pursuit of healthy populations through a combination of applied medical science (vaccination, for example) and various social policies and programs.[2] Some scholars also argue for a third phase, dating from the late 1970s, in which governments ceded ultimate responsibility (and thus prospective opprobrium) to the citizen-consumer.[3] While I address some themes of this latter phase in the final sections of this chapter, the connections between wartime and developments in mental health that I consider here sit squarely in the second phase. Indeed, in many ways the experience of mass warfare accelerated and expanded the remit of public health and, in so doing, solidified mental health as an object of government concern.

This interconnection is underscored by the fact that conceptualisations of psychiatric disorders and mental health during both world wars replicated a key preoccupation of public health policy during this period: the importance of prevention. Fostered by the mental hygiene movement, this ideal encompassed not only targeted therapeutic interventions but also policies that viewed individuals and families in hereditarian terms—a position in line with the eugenicist imperatives that circulated widely in the first half of the twentieth century. While historians have emphasised eugenics' broad agenda and political flexibility, at the core of the eugenicist worldview was the application of an 'evaluative logic' to reproduction—a racialised ideal achieved by preventing those designated unhealthy, diseased or otherwise damaged from reproducing.[4] As we will see, this had particularly sinister ramifications in a state like Nazi Germany, where sweeping racial and 'hereditary health' laws enacted in the 1930s not only mandated sterilisation for various groups on spurious medical, psychiatric, and racial grounds but also supplied justifications for the 'euthanasia' of children and adults deemed 'unworthy of life.' In this way, the Nazis vastly escalated and expanded the 'negative' eugenicist policies already in place in other nations, including the United States, where tens of thousands of people were sterilised under state statutes.[5]

As noted earlier, the mental hygiene movement also displayed a certain eugenicist sensibility that prefigured official reactions to the psychiatric problems caused by both world wars. The term 'hygiene' was itself implicative, an echo of the more sinister 'racial hygiene,' and conjured a systematised, scientific approach to 'preserving' or 'safeguarding' health, achieved by technocratic measures applied most vigorously to problem groups like the urban poor.[6] Here, again prevention was the watchword. For individuals with serious mental illness, this might mean prompt access to standard psychiatric help, including voluntary hospitalisation and effective aftercare upon release. But prevention also meant casting the net wider, enlisting several other categories of experts, including psychologists, sociologists, social workers, and welfare officers, to diagnose and combat the various social ills—alcoholism, prostitution, delinquency—that led to mental instability and illness. As outlined in the Introduction, in the United States mental hygiene was energetically promoted by the patient-turned-advocate Clifford Beers and the psychiatrist Adolf Meyer. While Beers was most concerned with the welfare of institutionalised patients, Meyer promoted mental hygiene as something more encompassing—not 'mere child psychiatry and a diluted general psychiatry,' but 'an intimate study and public education in favour of those factors which make for mental health in a positive, creative, and not merely a passive or mending way.'[7] In this way, mental hygiene reflected both Meyer's theoretical expansiveness and a broader Progressive-era interest in social reform.

Finally, growing medical and official interest in the psychological status of children reinforced the relationship between mental health and the health of the nation, insofar as the production of healthy 'normal' children was the ultimate preventative strategy. Here, there was a direct relationship with psychiatry's aetiological preoccupations. Psychiatry and the related psy disciplines had always been interested in childhood. Doctors who treated the hospitalised insane had long proposed that madness ran in families, and that early signs of hereditary insanity were observable in children.[8] Outside the asylum, the psychopathologies of childhood were central to psychoanalytic theorising.[9] This interest in children's psychological health coalesced with a broader medical interest in the health of children that had begun at the end of the nineteenth century and sought to improve both the bodies and minds of the working classes.[10] This tendency was inflated by the medical scrutiny of soldiers during the First World War. The ability to measure height, weight and (purportedly) intelligence promulgated extensive national literatures on the health of the male population and prompted further public health measures aimed at producing healthy children, such as adequate nutrition.[11] It also spawned increased scrutiny of parents and, with escalating intensity, the role of mothers in guaranteeing physically and mentally healthy offspring. In the first half of the twentieth century, 'scientific' childcare thus expanded to include not just correct nutrition, sanitation, and other forms of bodily care, but also the production of emotional health as understood through prevailing (and always changing) psychological paradigms. This national dimension justified the inroads of various forms of psychological expertise into the fields of child guidance, marriage guidance, and pedagogy, while also underscoring the importance of managing the psychopathologies of the adults on whom children depended.[12] Containing the psychological damage of wartime was one front in this effort.

The impact of mass warfare

As with medicine in general, the theory and practice of psychiatry were deeply impacted by the world wars, with both conflicts doing much to cement mental health as an individual objective and as a diffuse object of public policy. Mass warfare required psychiatrists and other clinicians to practise at scale; it also demonstrated the vulnerability of non-institutionalised people—and, most crucially, non-institutionalised men—to crippling psychological distress. Of course, the psychological effects of wartime were not confined to combatants, especially in the Second World War, when civilians were the explicit target of aerial bombardment, forced displacement, and genocide. But when it came to soldiers themselves, wartime posed searching questions about professional duty and individual conscience, encapsulated in the characteristic wartime conundrum: was the role of the clinician to treat the patient or to serve the nation? Demand for manpower meant that these objectives were not always in agreement. For example, a soldier exhibiting characteristic symptoms of shell shock during the 1916 Battle of the Somme might be best served therapeutically by evacuation from the horrors of the frontlines. But could his military unit afford him to be absent? Were military objectives best achieved by a psychiatric diagnosis or by disciplinary action? Did psychological distress constitute a war injury and thus furnish grounds for a pension? Negotiating largely irresolvable tensions between therapeutic necessity, discipline, and fiscal prudence would be an ongoing problem for military psychiatry in both world wars.

These problems were particularly pronounced in the First World War. One stark if uncommon outcome was the execution of soldiers who may have qualified for a diagnosis of 'shell shock' or similar conditions on the grounds of cowardice, desertion, and associated offences. In the British Army, around 350 men were executed during the conflict, a proportion of whom were likely suffering the psychological effects of trench warfare; in other national armies, the figures were likely much higher.[13] But for most soldiers suffering psychiatric symptoms, the outcome was less extreme. By the middle years of the war, it was clear to most armies on the Western Front that the terrors of attrition warfare—the relentless shell bombardments, the pointless charges into no man's land, the corpses hanging on the barbed wire—were producing psychiatric distress in many men. And, if no one could agree on the precise aetiology of what British personnel were now calling 'shell shock,' the sheer number of men made it a logistical problem above all else, reducible to a simple question: when a soldier suffering from characteristic symptoms presented to a regimental aid post, how should the presiding Medical Officer respond?[14] Evidence from the wave of psychiatric casualties that swamped the British on the Western Front in the middle of 1916 suggested that the reflex was to evacuate shell shock casualties to base hospitals, where soldiers either recovered and returned to the lines or, more concerningly, remained symptomatic and incapable of active duty. Under the guidance of Charles Myers, the psychologist who first used the term 'shell shock' in the medical literature, the British Army developed a new procedure to deal with these cases. Instead of evacuating them to the rear, soldiers would be sent to so-called 'rest centres' close to the frontlines, with a clear message that they were expected to recover and return to the fighting. Only the most serious cases would be sent to the base hospitals, and fewer still back to England, if these efforts of 'forward psychiatry' failed.[15]

This was prevention in action. An important principle thus emerged, one that was again expounded in the Second World War, but that also foretold a consequence of the emerging relationship between mass society and psychiatry: that increasingly, clinicians' primary concern would not be the institutionalised 'insane' but the walking wounded, people who were not 'mad' but distressed, often due to external circumstances. This type of patient did not necessarily require hospitalisation but could be treated with a combination of uncomplicated interventions—for the frontline soldier, sleep, food, fresh clothes, a gradual return to activity, and, if further help was required, attenuated versions of the newer talking therapies. If such intervention was swift and appropriate, the loss of function was temporary. In this way, psychiatry abetted the machinery of wartime: when men broke down, they were sent for repair. This was the more efficient and cost-effective approach, even if some of these men wore out eventually.

This is not to say that the First World War did not produce its share of what asylum doctors would have recognised as insanity. Some soldiers were clearly tipped into madness by the grim terror of their experiences, and in the interwar period, hundreds of 'forgotten lunatics' from the First World War remained in British psychiatric hospitals, many of them working-class soldiers subsisting on meagre pensions.[16] Periodic outcries about their condition competed with a broader official anxiety about the size of the pensions bill, a situation the authorities hoped to avoid in the next war. The Americans were particularly active in this regard, rolling out a vast 'pre-selection' scheme aimed at excluding men thought to be predisposed to psychiatric breakdown.[17] Even so, in the immediate aftermath of the Second World War, the Veterans' Administration struggled to cope with the sheer number of neuropsychiatric cases requiring treatment, which in 1946 comprised an estimated 60 % of all beds in the VA system and contributed to the uneasy sense that many veterans were irreparably damaged.[18] At the same time, this aggregation prompted important administrative changes to psychiatric terminology. While endemic imprecision had always frustrated clinicians in peacetime, it caused significant problems in the harried atmosphere of wartime, where standardised paperwork was vital for managing men within military bureaucracies. As head of Army Psychiatry in the United States, William Menninger developed the 'Medical 203' classification system, which expanded diagnostic categories to include circumstantially induced pathologies. This formed the basis of the first edition of the *Diagnostic and Statistical Manual* (DSM) published in 1952, supplanting the prior classification system (the *Statistical Manual for the Use of Institutions for the Insane*) designed for asylum populations.[19] This publication not only signalled the rising prestige of psychiatry within the medical landscape of post-war America but also fostered aspirations of making psychiatry and mental health universal.

The Vietnam War

If the world wars taught hard lessons about the practice of psychiatry at scale, clinical responses to the Vietnam War shifted emphasis to the more direct intersections of mental distress and politics. Much of this formed around questions of violence and its meanings. As with other professional associations, the Vietnam War was a persistently divisive issue for the APA over the course of the conflict, pitting anti-war psychiatrists against their more conservative peers. Though not universal, anti-war sentiment among the membership was widespread, and from the late sixties, the APA leadership experienced mounting pressure to publicly denounce the war on clinical grounds. Yet when the Board of Trustees finally did this in May 1971, characterising the war as promoting 'alienation, dehumanization, and divisiveness among the American people,' some members wrote to the *American Journal of Psychiatry* in protest.[20] One correspondent was 'disturbed at the idea of our association being used by some members as a platform for the expression of extreme left-wing political ideology'; it 'carries the prestige of psychiatry into what I consider an illegitimate area,' argued another.[21] Another was to ask searching questions about the relationship between professional duty and civic conscience, particularly as the draft escalated. Was issuing a draft exemption on a thin clinical pretext a justifiable act of civil disobedience or a dereliction of professional duty? In such cases, what were the long-term ramifications of designating a young man psychiatrically unfit?[22] Finally, how should anti-war psychiatrists regard the military psychiatrists who treated American soldiers for the psychiatric damage the war had inflicted? Wartime had always prompted tension between military necessity and psychiatrists' therapeutic impulses, but the conviction that the Vietnam War was unjust provoked outright criticism of military psychiatrists' claims to practise neutral medicine. As one disaffected former head of a neuropsychiatric unit put it, 'rigid and archaic military nosology' could not account for the many patients whose symptoms stemmed from their 'confrontation with the tragic absurdity' of killing or being killed in a 'meaningless military exercise' and whose 'entire being is devoted to extricating [themselves] from the situation.'[23] Another letter writer chided military psychiatrists for being 'too busy or too enamored with the task of secondary and tertiary prevention to ponder what primary prevention might have meant to the 13,000 Americans and the uncounted Vietnamese who have already died in the war.'[24]

Military psychiatrists exhibited their own scepticism towards the claims of anti-war psychiatrists, repeatedly pointing to low hospitalisation rates as evidence of soldiers' good morale and the military's careful planning.[25] But this argument became less tenable as the war progressed and the focus shifted from the psychiatric management of serving soldiers to the problems of veterans back in the United States. Critics pointed out that far from averting psychiatric harm, the 12-month tour meant that many soldiers broke down after discharge and were therefore never reflected in the military's casualty numbers.[26] Moreover, when veterans did show psychiatric symptoms, military and anti-war psychiatrists disagreed over the nature of their debility. The image of the Vietnam veteran as dangerously unstable and prone to violence was a staple of anti-war activism and reflected the conclusions of prominent anti-war clinicians like Chaim Shatan and Robert Jay Lifton, as well as older fears about returned soldiers as a vector for social unrest.[27] Shatan's 1972 article in the *New York Times*—the first to use 'Post-Vietnam Syndrome' as a clinical label—described the 'violent impulses against indiscriminate targets' provoked by counterinsurgency training and the difficulties of veterans in controlling these impulses in the face of 'ambivalence' back home.[28] Lifton also emphasised the 'bursts of anger' emanating from the veterans he encountered in stateside therapy groups, eruptions that underscored the 'rage and impulses towards violence' the Vietnam experience instilled.[29] In contrast, an official 1970 study of 50 returnees insinuated that the threat of violent veterans had been exaggerated for political reasons and that while 'the combat veteran may be more likely to talk about violence,' they were 'no more likely to behave violently.' Quoting from the seminal Second World War psychiatric treatise *Men Under Stress*, the authors reassured readers that '[n]ormal men nurtured by American civilization do not care to kill,' even when circumstances legitimated it.[30]

Yet evidence from Vietnam suggested otherwise. By the late 1960s, reporting on American activities in Vietnam had become more robust, fuelling public uneasiness about the expansion of the pacification program and the failure of the Tet Offensive—a sentiment emphatically compounded as revelations of the My Lai massacre emerged at the end of 1969.[31] In this context, the fear that Vietnam was turning 'ordinary American boys' into rage-filled killers intensified. As in previous wars, there was some acceptance that every army had its share of 'psychopaths' and 'sadists,' and there was at least one investigation into the childhoods of soldiers confessing to excessive violence for evidence of pathology.[32] Soldiers' illicit drug use was also of concern.[33] Most worrying, however, was the notion that for otherwise ordinary soldiers, the war had normalised the killing of defenceless civilians and replaced soldiers' guilt reactions with indifference. As the psychiatrist William Gault put it in a tellingly equivocal formulation, 'when soldiers observe or perpetuate slaughter, they often feel profoundly and enduringly guilty, and often they do not.'[34] Gault had spent 2 years at Fort Knox observing soldiers returning from Vietnam and emphasised the influence of situational factors in perpetuating violence against civilians: the perception of a pervasive but hidden enemy, the 'desperate trust and loyalty' that formed within combat units, the dehumanising of all Vietnamese by racist epithets. 'I am unwilling to attempt to draw any large lessons from my observations,' Gault concluded. 'But I think it safe to say that in Viet Nam a number of fairly ordinary young men have been psychologically ready to engage in slaughter and that moreover this readiness is by no means incomprehensible.'[35]

While this violence against civilians bolstered the moral arguments of the anti-war movement, the perpetrators themselves also served an important function for anti-war clinicians. Indeed, far from being reviled, the killer GI became both a symbol of the war's illegitimacy and its special brand of victim. In this regard, it was vital that the soldier who 'slaughtered' was not written off as a bad apple but instead viewed as the offshoot of a rotten tree—blameless, and capable of reform via skilled therapy. This was particularly true of the soldier who attended the group therapy sessions sponsored by the Veterans' Administration (VA) or the more informal 'rap' groups run by the Vietnam Veterans Against the War (VVAW), the organisation that convened the Winter Soldier hearings in Detroit in early 1971.[36] While this attitude unsettled some observers, who felt that overly solicitous therapists were offering veterans 'absolution' for war crimes, bestowing on veterans the double status of perpetrator-victim allowed theorists like Lifton to position them within a diagnostic lineage, as traumatised 'survivors.'[37] Throughout the 1950s and 1960s, a burgeoning literature on the suffering of Holocaust survivors had emphasised the persistence of victims' guilt feelings, due in part to an unconscious and defensive identification with their persecutors.[38] For Vietnam veterans, theorised Lifton, this identification, while no less anguished, was actual rather than symbolic, grounded in the veterans' dual identity, and manifested in the bursts of anger and ruminative guilt that characterised Post-Vietnam Syndrome.[39] From this vantage point, the ordinary American boys who razed Vietnamese villages and shot the inhabitants were themselves suffering from a psychic wound. As one veteran seeking admission to a VA psychiatric hospital put it, 'I have lost the sanctity of life.'[40]

In addition to making the morality of the war (though not, it is important to emphasise, the morality of individual soldiers) a clinical matter, Post-Vietnam Syndrome also rejected an exclusively interior model of psychic conflict, insisting on the primacy of actual events in evaluating psychiatric distress. The psychiatrist Stephen Howard, who in 1968 served as a battalion surgeon in Vietnam, emphasised the necessity of therapists who understood combat conditions, especially 'the ability and even desire to kill,' and who could resist the impulse to rationalise away 'anguish, horror, and guilt.' Like the suffering of Holocaust survivors, veterans' pain was caused by 'real acts and events,' not unconscious and largely symbolic conflicts.[41] Acknowledging this context had important practical effects. Just as sympathetic clinicians had argued to the West German reparations authorities that the psychological suffering of Jewish survivors stemmed not from claimants' pre-existing conditions but the singular nature of Nazi violence, anti-war clinicians posited that the Vietnam War had caused American soldiers to commit acts of moral trespass that were profoundly damaging to the psyche.[42] The government owed these men not just medical care but exculpation. To regard Post-Vietnam Syndrome as just another analogue of combat neurosis is therefore inaccurate. Instead, it was intended as both a diagnosis and a moral commentary on an unjust war in which the character of the animating violence held a central place.

Post-Vietnam Syndrome's tenure as a discrete disorder in public view was short-lived. From the mid-1970s consultations on the third edition of the DSM produced—cynics might say 'orchestrated'—sufficient clinical evidence for the creation of an encompassing diagnosis for patients suffering from ongoing traumatic stress. While there was initial resistance from clinicians who argued that veterans' symptoms were adequately explained by existing anxiety and substance abuse syndromes, anti-war clinicians like Lifton and Shatan were undeterred and played significant roles in collecting and then interpreting the clinical data that convinced Robert Spitzer, the initially sceptical chair of the DSM taskforce, of the validity of the disorder.[43] Post-Vietnam Syndrome and the survivor syndromes that preceded it coalesced in the more generalised diagnosis of post-traumatic stress disorder (PTSD), which debuted with the 1980 release of DSM-III. Whatever misgivings clinicians may have had about a loss of specificity were overtaken by pragmatic concerns. For veterans and other patients suffering from the long-term effects of traumatic events, PTSD gave them a legitimating diagnosis that could help facilitate access to medical care, especially as it recognised that symptoms could emerge long after the initial trigger.[44] And, in keeping with DSM-III's embrace of an empirically derived rather than abstractly theorised classification model, it removed some of the stigma of the highly subjective, psychoanalytically informed diagnostic schemas that regarded a patient's defective personality as the main driver of psychiatric illness.[45] This shift in focus from the patient to the precipitating event essentially reversed the diagnostic burden of proof, implying that certain catastrophic events would damage almost anyone.[46]

Yet there were costs to such an approach. As its critics have noted, PTSD is not only neutral when it comes to the role of patients' personalities in fostering psychiatric symptoms but also ecumenical in its ascription of traumatic effects. In this sense, while the sufferings of Holocaust survivors or Vietnam veterans might be characteristic, they are not constitutive. Once a certain threshold of seriousness is reached, PTSD is inclusive, its diagnostic criteria satisfied equally by a Holocaust survivor, a victim of a serious car accident, a target of an armed robbery, and, ultimately, a villager whose family was massacred in a pacification raid and the GIs who did the killing.[47] It is not just that PTSD 'amoralised' or 'decontextualised' trauma, as its critics have claimed, but that it also diverted scrutiny from the specific character of the violence underlying patients' symptoms.[48] In doing so, it reduced the possibilities for incorporating socio-political commentary into clinical work. Therapy no longer required a moral accounting, nor an examination of the institutions and actions that had made the violence possible. Clinicians worked to erase patients' symptoms with therapy and, increasingly, medication. Over time, these treatments were written into military budgets as operational expenditure, making PTSD a cost but not a critique of war. Rising contemporary interest in the concept of 'moral injury' suggests that many service personnel and veterans find PTSD to be an unsatisfactory framework for understanding their experiences, particularly if they have participated in the morally contentious wars in Iraq and Afghanistan.[49]

If militaries' acceptance of PTSD worked to depoliticise the psychological damage wrought by war, in other settings PTSD and the broader field of trauma theory made other kinds of psychological suffering visible. During the 1980s and 1990s, work by feminist clinicians such as Judith Lewis Herman reinscribed victims of sexual violence, domestic violence, and child abuse as trauma survivors, arguing that damage could accrue over long periods, that symptoms could be dormant for long periods and—controversially—that individuals might unknowingly suppress traumatic memories as a survival strategy.[50] In these formulations, traumatic experience appeared as a common occurrence, particularly for women, often fostered in childhood, demonstrable via the Adverse Childhood Experience scoring system, and thus a means of political critique.[51] The concept of intergenerational trauma, and allied concepts like historical and racial trauma, serves a similarly important function for advocates of reparative justice. Originally understood as a form of psychodynamic dysfunction in the families of Holocaust survivors, intergenerational trauma is now increasingly proposed as an epigenetically mediated form of inherited stress, and thus applicable to the descendants of people subjected to historical violence and mistreatment, including the enslaved and the colonised, over and above the contemporary stressors produced by racism and socioeconomic disadvantage.[52] At the same time, the reconceptualisation of intergenerational trauma in these biomedical terms could prove problematic for constituencies seeking to articulate the magnitude of historical wrongs while also avoiding malign imputations of permanent pathology.

New explanatory models of intergenerational trauma are one example of the way trauma theory has adapted to psychiatry's reigning biomedical framework. More broadly, there have also been calls to reframe PTSD as a 'systemic illness,' one that transcends traditional medical specialities, a position supported by clinicians' turn towards biological and 'neuro' interventions like the psychopharmaceuticals, REMD and NLP techniques discussed in the previous chapter.[53] These developments suggest that trauma can now be posited as both culturally and individually pervasive: rife in the population and in traumatised bodies themselves. Political claims about mental health also have purchase here. In his bestselling *The Body Keeps the Score*, trauma clinician Bessel van der Kolk suggests that trauma is 'arguably the greatest threat to our national well-being,' a situation that can only be remedied by 'a massive effort to help children and adults learn to deal with the fear, rage, and collapse' that are 'the predictable consequences of having been traumatized.'[54]

Psychiatry and state repression

The ructions in the APA during the Vietnam War foreshadowed another controversy about professional ethics in operational settings: the involvement of American psychologists in the 'enhanced' interrogation techniques used on inmates of the Guantanamo Bay detention centre and other sites at the height of the War on Terror. Whereas the APA and the American Medical Association (AMA) had restricted their members' participation in these practices as contrary to their healing oaths, a mixture of patriotism and financial inducements fostered a warmer relationship between the leadership of the American Psychological Association (ApA) and national security officials. This resulted in what one critic characterised as a kind of 'motivated ignorance,' in which the prospect of prestige and funding overruled ethical concerns.[55] In October 2005, the ApA President Ronald F. Levant travelled to Guantanamo Bay with other observers, a trip he regarded as 'an important opportunity for the Association to provide input on the question of how psychologists can play an appropriate and ethical role in national security investigations.'[56] Soon emissaries from the CIA and the Department of Defence were questioning experts like Martin Seligman, famous for developing the concept of 'learned helplessness,' on how to best prepare American POWs for the rigours of capture—knowledge they also applied to the interrogation of detainees in American custody.[57] According to an investigation commissioned by the ApA's Board of Directors in response to significant internal dissent and public pressure, the ApA leadership also cooperated with US Department of Defense officials to produce ethics guidelines that did not preclude psychologists' participation in interrogations. The investigation concluded that the main motivation for this cooperation was to 'curry favour with DoD,' as well as 'create a good public-relations response, and to keep the growth of psychology unrestrained in this area.'[58]

While the disputes over American clinicians' involvement in the Vietnam War and the War on Terror are comparatively recent controversies, the history of psychiatry and adjacent disciplines' involvement with repressive regimes across the course of the twentieth century suggests that psychiatry is capable of fostering both collusion and resistance to authoritarianism. Perhaps the most notorious example is Nazi Germany. It is no surprise that Nazism was reflexively hostile to the 'Jewish science' of psychoanalysis, and that Jewish and anti-fascist analysts in Germany and then Austria soon perceived their lives to be in danger. After the Anschluss, the elderly Freud and his immediate family went into exile in London, the most prominent example of the émigré clinicians who left the continent before the war. (Not so four of Freud's sisters who, unable to leave Vienna, died in the Holocaust.)[59] A small number of racially vetted psychoanalysts colluded with the regime, participating in a de-Judaised, Nazified form of psychotherapy that emphasised the psychic importance of serene integration into the *Volksgemeinschaft*.[60]

The situation for institutional psychiatrists was different. Indeed, for clinicians who supported the regime or were willing to compromise with it, there were new professional opportunities as the state 'coordinated' the profession and put it to work on its racial projects. This was not just about 'de-Judaising' Germany but purifying the Aryan race itself, meaning there was no place for the mentally defective in the new Germany. Initially, the Nazis persecuted the mentally ill and the physically and intellectually disabled by way of marriage proscriptions and compulsory sterilisation—the latter not unfamiliar to the Western democracies, as we have seen.[61] But as with other aspects of Nazi racial policy, these measures escalated rapidly, especially after the declaration of war in September 1939. The first targets were infants and young children institutionalised due to physical and mental disabilities. Between October 1939 and the end of the war, some 5000 children were murdered, usually by lethal overdose, in a secretive (although not unknown) child 'euthanasia' project coordinated by the Führer Chancellery. This predated the *Aktion T4* program that began in January 1940 and saw institutionalised adults gassed to death in six purpose-built facilities in Germany and Austria. While concern about public disquiet called an official halt to this centralised killing in August 1941, for the rest of the war euthanasia wards in individual institutions continued to murder disabled adults and psychiatric patients via lethal overdoses and starvation. An estimated 70,000 adults were killed during the centralised 'euthanasia' phase; perhaps one hundred thousand more were murdered during the 'decentralised' period.[62]

Psychiatrists, neurologists, and other clinicians colluded in this mass murder out of ideological conviction or for professional advancement, as well as for access to research material; the Clinic for Psychiatry and Neurology at Heidelberg University and the Brandenburg-Görden State Hospital were two organisations that regarded the euthanasia program as a research opportunity.[63] Other moral compromises continue to generate controversy. In Vienna, the physician Hans Asperger (of 'Asperger's syndrome' fame) and his staff were careful to protect the children in his Paediatric Clinic from the child euthanasia program. Yet Asperger also appears to have participated in that same program in a modified way, on at least two occasions sending a child to the Am Spiegelgrund clinic where euthanasia murders were carried out. A sympathetic interpretation is that Asperger was unclear on what exactly was happening in these institutions and that because the Nazis always doubted Asperger's loyalty, these shows of cooperation kept his clinic children safe. A bleaker view is that Asperger, like many of his colleagues, *could* countenance the killing of 'unworthy' children, just not the highly intelligent 'little professors' in his clinic.[64]

The mass murder of psychiatric patients and other institutionalised people is closely linked to the Nazis' other exterminatory projects. Historians of the Holocaust such as Henry Friedlander have argued that the murder of institutionalised children and adults did not just test German public opinion on state-sanctioned mass killing but also produced practical knowledge about the infrastructure and expertise required for genocide.[65] The murder of patients by clinical personnel in reputed medical settings thus fed the wider machinery of extermination in several ways. Inside Germany, the 'euthanasia' gassing facilities were repurposed to kill sick and exhausted concentration camp inmates and, during the war, forced labourers ill with tuberculosis and nursing home residents taking up hospital beds. As the war expanded in the east, euthanasia personnel were redeployed to extermination camps in Poland. Finally, the euthanasia programs within Germany pre-empted the genocide of Europe's Jewish communities by targeting German-Jewish patients in institutions on racial rather than medical grounds. Few remained alive to be deported eastwards. In Eastern Europe, too, some psychiatric hospitals housing Jewish patients were simply 'cleared' during liquidation actions: in August 1942, for example, around 100 patients at the Zofiówka Hospital near Warsaw were summarily shot.[66] Such atrocities were in addition to the general risks of starvation and neglect for vulnerable institutionalised patients. In occupied France, for example, up to 45,000 asylum inmates are thought to have died from starvation during the war.[67]

While the situation in Nazi Germany was extreme, in the Soviet Union psychiatry was also bent to state ends. Western scholarship on Soviet psychiatry has tended to emphasise two themes: first, its Pavlovian rather than Freudian bent and, second, its use against dissidents (an issue that came to prominence in the 1970s).[68] While both characterisations are accurate to a degree, they do not tell the full story of Soviet psychiatry, which at least until the Stalin period had much in common with the psychiatry practised in Europe and the Anglo-American world. From the end of the nineteenth century, Russian clinicians forged strong transnational connections with practitioners in Europe and in the Anglo-American world. War and revolution in the first decade of the twentieth century disrupted but did not eliminate these links; nor did they destroy the international sensibility crucial to the circulation of psychiatric knowledge during this period. Indeed, throughout the 1920s the government actively supported a Soviet psychiatry that was transnational in outlook, albeit increasingly orientated toward state ends—one also that emphasised the importance of extraneous environment factors, the possibility of rehabilitation, and the corresponding virtues of early intervention.[69] Of course, much of this was ideologically congruent. In the years after the Revolution and Civil War, the Communist Party was particularly receptive to psychiatrists who claimed that conditions of extreme inequality caused nervous disorder and general ill health, and that experts were needed to remediate the trauma of more recent war and deprivation, especially the damage done to children.[70] For their part, Soviet psychiatrists, under-resourced like their counterparts elsewhere, relished the possibility of increased funding and professional advancement.

This focus on external factors was in keeping with developments in broader psychiatric thought and practice in the interwar period. For most of the 1920s, Soviet clinicians continued to participate in international conferences and exchanges, receiving foreign visitors and sending their students to train in foreign universities. Advances in psychiatry during this period were 'fruits of exchanges and borrowings that were multidirectional, reformulated into a project that was new and coherent.'[71] Soviet clinicians' embrace of the mental hygiene movement is a case in point. Leading figures like Lev Rozenshtein had read Adolf Meyer and shared his views on the multiple factors that might cause mental distress. Meyer would eventually visit the Soviet Union on a lecture tour in June 1933. Soviet psychiatrists also espoused the value of early intervention in non-institutional settings. Like their counterparts in the United States, Soviet clinicians believed that there was a deep well of unrecognised pathology in the community at large, and that shifting clinical efforts from the asylum to the general population would ultimately relieve pressure on the overcrowded institutions that cared for the seriously mentally ill. The development of outpatient facilities in the 1920s was the key means of accomplishing this and an initiative that chimed with the Bolshevik vision of public health as a vehicle for modernisation and surveillance. Outpatient clinics were established in major cities, prime among them the State Health Centre of Neurology and Psychiatry (later the Institute for Prophylaxis in Neurology and Psychiatry) opened in Moscow in 1924 and overseen by Rozenshtein. (As in other jurisdictions, the countryside remained under-served.)[72]

As with so much else, the official attitude towards psychiatry hardened under Stalin. The 1932 campaign to purify philosophy soon encompassed most areas of inquiry, including research into mental disorders, so that conceptual models were now required to reflect 'correct' Soviet doctrines and to expend greater efforts in supporting the industrialisation drive. Proponents of mental hygiene were attacked for undermining these efforts, for championing Western ideas and for diverting resources away from psychiatric hospitals and the seriously mentally ill.[73] Other strands of psychiatric theory and practice were also jeopardised as the Stalinist terror grew. Psychoanalysis, which had been tolerated by the early Bolsheviks despite scepticism about its compatibility with Marxism, was banned outright in 1930.[74] Of course, at the height of the Great Purges, any kind of 'talking therapy' entailed extreme risk, and many psychoanalysts fled to the West or stopped practising during this period. Sabina Spielrein, an early patient of Jung's and by the interwar period an important theorist in her own right, went into exile in Rostov and was murdered there, along with her daughters, in the Einzsatgruppen massacre at the Zmeyevskaya Ravine in August 1942.[75]

Psychiatry remained politically useful in the Soviet Union after the Stalinist period. Under Khrushchev (1953–1964) the state relaxed its surveillance and persecution of dissidents, many of whom were allowed to return from exile. In the psychiatric sphere, the adoption of chlorpromazine signalled an openness to new developments.[76] Under Brezhnev (1964–1982), however, a new generation of dissidents was subjected to renewed forms of juridical control, including more stringent vagrancy laws and incarceration in psychiatric hospitals on the grounds of specious diagnoses, including the notorious 'sluggish schizophrenia.'[77] Human rights literature in the West had much to say about the injustice done to these political opponents—the case of mathematician Leonid Plyushch made headlines around the world—but less about the plight of the psychiatrically ill themselves, whose rights were also compromised by maltreatment.[78] If the practice of psychiatry in the Soviet Union was at once more repressive *and* more heterogeneous than surface accounts disclose, scholarship on psychiatry in Eastern Europe suggests even greater departures from the caricature of inflexible Pavlovianism. For those clinicians able to travel, there remained opportunities for transnational exchange with colleagues in the West, just as clinicians from Western Europe, Britain, and the United States were sometimes visitors to their colleagues in parts of Eastern Europe. Practitioners in non-aligned Yugoslavia played a particularly important role as intermediaries between East and West, a position replicated in other medical fields.[79]

The persistence of these international links, as well as the diversity of theories and practices on the ground, underscore psychiatry's lack of innate political categories. Argentina offers another example of this dynamic, albeit one more distinctly confined to the position of psychoanalytic psychology in a repressive regime. In Argentina, psychoanalysis followed a different trajectory to the Anglo-American world, installing itself in academic psychology rather than psychiatry and incorporating a significant Lacanian influence.[80] Yet its extraordinary position in Argentinian public health infrastructure—an oft-quoted figure is that one in every 200 residents of Buenos Aires is a psychoanalytic psychologist, and that even Pope Francis has gone to therapy—is the result not of persistent state investment but the discipline's mid-century repression.[81] Psychoanalysis was antithetical to Perónism and the conservative Catholicism of its support base, but it nevertheless flourished in university psychology programs from the mid-1950s until the 1966 coup d'état, when the military assumed control of the universities.[82] Individual theoreticians and clinicians were then expelled or went into exile; others were murdered during the Dirty War (1974–1983); much of the remainder retreated into the private sphere; a small number of dissident analysts worked with other opponents of the regime, including those whose family members had been 'disappeared.'[83] Yet because the regime did not regard psychoanalysis as an especially worrisome locus of resistance, this undercut any incipient radicalism—so much so that the Lacanism that took hold in the 1980s 'was completely purged of any Marxist tendencies.'[84] According to one commentator, the history of Argentinian psychoanalysis thus 'contradicts the popular idea that psychoanalysis can only flourish in free and democratic environments,' demonstrating that 'psychoanalysis, like any other system of thought, can be appropriated and used in different ways and for contradictory purposes.'[85]

Conclusion

The relationship between states and psychiatry and other psy disciplines solidified across the twentieth century, propelled by states' increasing interest in public health and by the usefulness of psychiatric knowledge during wartime. In Anglo-American contexts, the large numbers of psychiatric casualties resulting from the First and Second World Wars produced a change in the prototypical patient seeking treatment for mental distress—a move away from the hospitalised insane towards otherwise 'normal' patients suffering from affective distress. The formulation of the post-traumatic stress disorder (PTSD) diagnosis in the aftermath of the Vietnam War and the proliferation of trauma theory more generally also confirm the potentially diffuse effects of psychiatry's interest in the mental effects of war. Finally, the controversy over American psychiatrists' involvement in the Vietnam War, and the important role of anti-war clinicians in publicising the mental suffering of Vietnam veterans, highlights the thorough imbrication of psychiatric knowledge with politics. Just as psychiatry could be mobilised in opposition to the Vietnam War, so too could it be instrumentalised by repressive states. The history of the relationship between states and psychiatry thus suggests that psychiatry and ideas about mental health more generally can serve diverse political ends. While particularly amenable to instrumentalisation by the powerful, psychiatry may also provide less powerful actors with a language of resistance. This ambivalence is evident not just within nation states but in the history of colonisation and globalisation, as the next chapter sets out.

Notes

1 Alison Bashford, *Imperial Hygiene: A Critical History of Colonialism, Nationalism and Public Health* (Palgrave Macmillan, 2003), 1; for isolation and confinement of the sick in an urban setting see Matthew Newson Kerr, *Contagion, Isolation, and Biopolitics in Victorian London* (Palgrave, 2018).

2 For historical overviews see George Rosen, *A History of Public Health* (MD Publications, 1958), Dorothy Porter, *Health, Civilization and the State: A History of Public Health from Ancient to Modern Times* (Routledge, 1999), and Sophy Bergenheim, Johan Edman, Johannes Kananen and Merle Wessel, 'Introduction', in *Conceptualising Public Health: Historical and Contemporary Struggles Over Key Concepts* (Routledge, 2018), 1–17.
3 See for example Nike Ayo, 'Understanding Health Promotion in a Neoliberal Climate and the Making of Health Conscious Citizens', *Critical Public Health* 22, no. 1 (2012): 99–105.
4 Alison Bashford and Philippa Levine, 'Introduction: Eugenics and the Modern World', in *The Oxford Handbook of the History of Eugenics*, ed. Alison Bashford and Philippa Levine (Oxford University Press, 2010), 3–4.
5 See Molly Ladd-Taylor, *Fixing the Poor: Eugenic Sterilization and Child Welfare in the Twentieth Century* (Johns Hopkins University Press, 2020), particularly 227–30 on the challenges of obtaining accurate statistics.
6 Randall M. Packard, *A History of Global Health: Interventions into the Lives of Other People* (Johns Hopkins University Press, 2016), 61.
7 Adolf Meyer, 'The Fourteenth Maudsley Lecture: British Influences in Psychiatry and Mental Hygiene', *Journal of Mental Science* 79 (1933): 458.
8 See Theodore M. Porter, *Genetics in the Madhouse: The Unknown History of Human Heredity* (Princeton University Press, 2018).
9 For an overview see Pierre Geissmann and Claudine Geissmann, *A History of Child Psychoanalysis* (Routledge, 1998).
10 See the edited collection *Children's Health Issues in Historical Perspective*, ed. Cheryl Krasnick Warsh and Veronica Strong-Boag (Wilfrid Laurier University Press, 2005) and in *In the Name of the Child: Health and Welfare, 1880–1940*, ed. Roger Cooter (Routledge, 1992).
11 See for example Ina Zweiniger-Bargielowska, *Managing the Body: Beauty, Health and Fitness in Britain, 1880–1939* (Oxford University Press, 2010), particularly 193–235.
12 On scientific mothering in the United States see Rima D. Apple, *Perfect Motherhood: Science and Childrearing in America* (Rutgers University Press, 2006); for the British context see Shual Bar-Haim, *The Maternalists: Psychoanalysis, Motherhood, and the British Welfare State* (University of Philadelphia Press, 2021).
13 For an overview see John Hughes-Wilson, 'Pardons for All', *Royal United Services Institute for Defence Studies* 151, no. 5 (2006): 56–59. For estimated numbers of executions per nation, see Steven R. Welch, 'Military Justice', in *1914–1918 Online: International Encyclopedia of the First World War* (2014), https://encyclopedia.1914-1918-online.net/article/military_justice.
14 On shell shock and its various meanings see Tracy Loughran, *Shell-Shock and Medical Culture in First World War Britain* (Cambridge University Press, 2017); for its relationship to the broader idea of 'shock' see Stefanos Geroulanos and Todd Meyers, *The Human Body in the Age of Catastrophe: Brittleness, Integration, Science, and the Great War* (University of Chicago Press, 2018), 34–77.
15 On 'forward psychiatry' see Ben Shephard, *A War of Nerves: Soldiers and Psychiatrists in the Twentieth Century* (Harvard University Press, 2001), 53–71 and Edgar Jones and Simon Wessely, *Shell Shock to PTSD: Military Psychiatry from 1900 to the Gulf War* (Psychology Press, 2005), 24–31.
16 Peter Barham, *Forgotten Lunatics of the Great War* (Yale University Press, 2007).
17 Naoko Wake, 'The Military, Psychiatry, and "Unfit" Soldiers, 1939–1942', *Journal of the History of Medicine and Allied Sciences* 62, no. 4 (2007): 461–94.
18 On the pressures on VA hospitals see Daniel Blain, 'Some Essentials in National Mental Health Planning', *BMC* (November 1946): 180–81; on concerns about returning veterans, see Martin Halliwell, 'Going Home: World War II and Demobilization' in *Therapeutic Revolutions*, 17–47.
19 Allan V. Horwitz, *DSM: A History of Psychiatry's Bible* (Johns Hopkins University Press, 2021), 19–23.

20 'Official Actions: Highlights of the 124th Annual Meeting', *American Journal of Psychiatry* (hereafter '*AJP*') 128, no. 1 (1971): 137–40, 139.
21 See letters from W. Johnson and H. Corral, 'Statements about Viet Nam: APA's Role', *AJP* 130, no. 6 (1973): 721–22; J. Gunderson (ed.), 'Letters to the Editor: Viet Nam: The Board of Trustees Steps Out of Bounds', *AJP* 130, no. 5 (1973): 610.
22 I.M. Frank and F.S. Hoedemaker, 'The Civilian Psychiatrist and the Draft', *AJP* 127, no. 4 (1970): 497–502; J.A. Moskowitz, 'On Drafting the Psychiatric "Draft" Letter', *AJP* 128, no. 1 (1971): 69–72.
23 T. Maier, 'The Army Psychiatrist—An Adjunct to the System of Social Control', *AJP* 126, no. 7 (1970): 1039.
24 E.C. Levin, 'Evading the Realities of War?', *AJP* 124, no. 8 (1968): 1138. Levin was responding to R.E. Strange and R.J. Arthur's article published the previous year: 'Hospital Ship Psychiatry in a War Zone', *AJP* 124, no. 3 (1967): 281–86.
25 For characteristic assessments see E.M. Colbach and M.D. Parrish, 'Army Mental Health Activities in Vietnam: 1965–1970', *Bulletin of the Menninger Clinic* 34, no. 6 (1970): 333–42; W.J. Tiffany and W. Allerton, 'Army Psychiatry in the Mid-60s', *AJP* 123, no. 7 (1967): 810–18; and W.J. Tiffany, 'The Mental Health of Army Troops in Viet Nam', *AJP* 123, no. 12 (1967): 1585–86.
26 See S. Howard, 'The Vietnam Warrior: His Experience, and Implications for Psychotherapy', *AJP* 30, no. 1 (1976): 121–35, specifically 130–31.
27 This fear was particularly pronounced in the interwar period; for an overview see M. Edele and R. Gerwarth, 'The Limits of Demobilisation: Global Perspectives on the Aftermath of the Great War', *Journal of Contemporary History* 50, no. 1 (2015): 3–14.
28 C.F. Shatan, 'Post-Vietnam Syndrome', *The New York Times*, 6 May 1972, 35.
29 R.J. Lifton, *Home from the War: Vietnam Veterans—Neither Victims nor Executioners* (Simon and Schuster, 1973), 137.
30 Cdr. R.E. Strange and Capt. D.E. Brown, 'Home From the War: A Study of Psychiatric Problems in Viet Nam Returnees', *AJP* 127, no. 4 (1970): 488–92, 492; R.R. Grinker and J.P. Spiegel, *Men Under Stress* (Blakiston, 1945).
31 See K. Oliver, *The My Lai Massacre in American History and Memory* (Manchester University Press, 2006), particularly 20–25 on the shift in reporting culture. On the massacre as a 'crisis of American mythography' see R. Slotkin, *Gunfighter Nation: The Myth of the Frontier in Twentieth Century America* (HarperPerennial, 1993), 578–91.
32 J. Yager, 'Personal Violence in Infantry Combat', *Archives of General Psychiatry* (hereafter '*Arch Gen Psych*') 32, no. 2 (1975): 257–61. In a subsequent study Yager proposed that certain soldiers seemed to be 'violence-prone' before, during and after combat: 'Postcombat Violent Behaviour in Psychiatrically Maladjusting Soldiers', *Arch Gen Psych* 33, no. 11 (1976): 1332–35.
33 See for example Jerome Char, 'Drug Abuse in Viet Nam', *AJP* 129, no. 4 (1972): 463–65; see also Lucas Richert, *Break on Through: Radical Psychiatry and the American Counterculture* (The MIT Press, 2019), 17–18.
34 W.B. Gault, 'Some Remarks on Slaughter', *AJP* 128, no. 4 (1971): 451.
35 Gault, 'Some Remarks', 451–52 and 454. For another account of the war turning hitherto 'normal' young men into killers see H.P. Langner, 'The Making of a Murderer', *AJP* 127, no. 7 (1971): 950–53.
36 For a detailed if somewhat morally detached account of the pacification program, see R.A. Hunt, *Pacification: The American Struggle for Vietnam's Hearts and Minds* (Westview Press, 1995). On the Winter Soldier hearings see Oliver, *The My Lai Massacre*, 109.
37 See the discussion in Ben Shephard, *A War of Nerves: Soldiers and Psychiatrists in the Twentieth Century* (Harvard University Press, 2001), 373–76. For an account of how this position might have contributed to sympathy for Lieutenant Calley, another 'ordinary American boy', during his court martial, see Oliver, *The My Lai Massacre*, 127–31.
38 For an overview of this literature see Ruth Leys, *From Guilt to Shame: Auschwitz and After* (Princeton University Press, 2007), particularly 32–63.

39 See Lifton, *Home from the War*, 36–37, where he describes the perpetrators of the My Lai massacre as 'survivors.' For his previous formulations of survivorhood, which extrapolate the experience of survivors of the Hiroshima bombing to humanity in general, see R.J. Lifton, *Death in Life: Survivors of Hiroshima* (University of North Carolina Press, 1991), 479: 'we are all survivors of Hiroshima and, in our imaginations, of future nuclear holocaust.' See also Shephard, *War of Nerves*, 360–61.
40 Yager, 'Personal Violence in Infantry Combat', 258.
41 Howard, 'The Vietnam Warrior', 132.
42 On the role of the West German compensation process in prompting the development of survivor guilt, see Leys, *From Guilt to Shame*, 32–36 and Herzog, *Cold War Freud: Psychoanalysis in an Age of Catastrophe* (Cambridge University Press, 2017), 94–106.
43 See Alan Young, *The Harmony of Illusions: Inventing Post-Traumatic Stress Disorder* (Princeton University Press, 1995), 107–16 and Hannah Decker, *The Making of DSM-III: A Diagnostic Manual's Conquest of American Psychiatry* (Oxford University Press, 2013), 274–75.
44 Clinicians in Oregon, for example, reported an 'unprecedented' increase in claims for VA benefits beginning October 1980, when the VA recognised 'delayed type' PTSD as grounds for compensation: R.M. Atkinson, et al., 'Assessment of Viet Nam Veterans for Posttraumatic Stress Disorder in Veterans Administration Disability Claims', *AJP* 139, no. 9 (1982): 1118–21.
45 See Young, *Harmony of Illusions*, 94–102.
46 Didier Fassin and Richard Rechtmann have referred to this as 'the consecration of the event': see Fassin and Rechtmann, *The Empire of Trauma: An Inquiry into the Condition of Victimhood*, trans. by Rachel Gomme (Princeton University Press, 2009), 84–87.
47 Ruth Leys argues that this commodious tendency might make trauma 'debased currency': *Trauma: A Genealogy* (University of Chicago Press, 2000), 2. Fassin and Rechtman make a similar point about the effects of grouping many 'signifieds' into a single 'signifier': *Empire of Trauma*, 277.
48 See Herzog, *Cold War Freud*, 113–22. In slight contrast, Fassin and Rechtmann argue that PTSD has fostered an 'unprecedented ability to talk about—and hence to experience—the violence of the world', but that this is achieved by 'subsuming' categories of violence into a single construct: *The Empire of Trauma*, 275–84.
49 For a discussion of this concept see Kenneth MacLeish, 'On "Moral Injury": Psychic Fringes and War Violence', *History of the Human Sciences* 31, no. 2 (2018): 128–46.
50 Judith Lewis Herman, *Trauma and Recovery* (Basic Books, 2001).
51 On the origins of the Adverse Childhood Experiences (ACE) study see Vincent J. Felitti, 'Origins of the ACE Study', *American Journal of Preventative Medicine* 56, no. 6 (2019): 787–89.
52 See Rachel Yehuda and Amy Lehrner, 'Intergenerational Transmission of Trauma Effects: Putative Role of Epigenetic Mechanisms', *World Psychiatry* 17, no. 3 (2018): 243–57. For an overview addressing the question of whether historical or racial trauma ought to be understood literally or metaphorically see Joseph P. Gone, 'The Impact of Historical Trauma on Health Outcomes for Indigenous Populations in the USA and Canada: A Systematic Review', *American Psychologist* 74, no. 1 (2019): 20–35.
53 The link with cardiovascular disease is proposed to be particularly strong: see David S. Krantz, et al., 'Post Traumatic Stress Disorder as a Systematic Disorder: Pathways to Cardiovascular Disease', *Health Psychology* 41, no. 10 (2022): 651–62 and Alexander C. McFarlane, 'Post-Traumatic Stress Disorder Is a Systemic Illness, Not a Mental Disorder: Is Cartesian Dualism Dead?', *MJA* 206, no. 6 (2017): 248–49.
54 Bessel Van Der Kolk, *The Body Keeps the Score: Mind, Brain and Body in the Transformation of Trauma* (Penguin, 2014), 348. Van Der Kolk also emphasises the ACE findings: 143–47.
55 Dan Aalbers, 'The Hoffman Report in Historical Context: A Study in Denial', *History of the Human Sciences* 35, no. 5 (2022): 27.

56 Ronald F. Levant, 'Visit to the U.S. Joint Task Force Station at Guantanamo Bay: A First Person Account', *Military Psychology* 19 (2007): 2.

57 Seligman continues to defend his contact with national security officials, arguing that 'unfashionable as it is, I strongly believe that when in doubt we should err on the side of helping our soldiers and our nation': Martin Seligman, 'The Hoffman Report, the Central Intelligence Agency, and the Defense of the Nation: A Personal View', *Health Psychology Open* 5, no. 2 (2018): 8.

58 'Report to the Special Committee of the Board of Directors of the American Psychological Association: Independent Review Relating to APA Ethics Guidelines, National Security Interrogations, and Torture', 2015, 9.

59 For Freud in exile see the edited collection *Freud and the Émigré: Austrian Émigrés, Exiles and the Legacy of Psychoanalysis in Britain, 1930s—1970s*, ed. Elana Shapira and Daniela Finzi (Springer, 2020).

60 See the accounts in Geoffrey Cocks, *Psychotherapy in the Third Reich: The Göring Institute* (Transaction Publishers, 1997) and Laura Sokolowsky, *Psychoanalysis Under Nazi Occupation* (Routledge, 2021).

61 For an overview of these laws see Henry Friedlander, *The Origins of Nazi Genocide: From Euthanasia to the Final Solution* (University of North Carolina Press, 1995), 42–56.

62 See Friedlander, *Origins of Nazi Genocide*; Michael S. Bryant, *Confronting the 'Good Death': Nazi Euthanasia on Trial, 1945–1953* (University Press of Colorado, 2005), 19–62; and Patricia Heberer, 'The Nazi "Euthanasia" Program', in *Routledge History of the Holocaust*, ed. Jonathan C. Friedman (Routledge, 2011). For an example of how unofficial euthanasia continued after August 1941, see Susan Benedict and Tessa Chelouche, 'Meseritz-Obrawalde: A "Wild Euthanasia" Hospital of Nazi Germany', *History of Psychiatry* 19, no. 1 (2008): 68–76.

63 Friedlander, *Origins of the Nazi Genocide*, 140. On the fate of brain specimens taken from some victims, see Paul Weindling, et al., 'The Problematic Legacy of Victim Specimens from the Nazi Era: Identifying the Persons Behind the Specimens at the Max Planck Institutes for Brain Research and of Psychiatry', *Journal of the History of the Neurosciences* 32, no. 2 (2023): 218–39.

64 The case for Asperger's complicity is set out in Herwig Czech, 'Hans Asperger, National Socialism, and "Race Hygiene" in Nazi-era Vienna', *Molecular Autism* 9, no. 29 (2018): 1–43 and 'Response to "Non-complicit: Revisiting Hans Asperger's Career in Nazi-era Vienna', *JADD* 49 (2019), 3883–87 . For defences of Asperger see Ernst Tatzer, Werner Maleczek and Franz Waldhauser, 'An Assessment of What Hans Asperger Knew About Child Euthanasia in Vienna During the Nazi Occupation', *Acta Paediatrica* 112, no. 5 (2023): 1109–19; Dean Falk, 'Non-complicit: Revisiting Hans Asperger's Career in Nazi-era Vienna', *Journal of Austism and Developmental Disorders* (hereafter '*JADD*') 50 (2020): 2573–84; and 'More on Asperger's Career: A Reply to Czech', *JADD* 49 (2019): 3877–82.

65 Friedlander, *Origins of the Nazi Genocide*, 11.

66 For the fate of Jewish psychiatric patients in Germany and on the Eastern Front, see Friedlander, *Origins of the Nazi Genocide*, 268–87 and Kamila Uzarczyk, '"Schluss Mit Der Rassenschande!" From Separation to Extermination: The Fate of Jewish Mentally Ill Patients in Germany and Occupied Poland, 1939–42', in *Recognizing the Past in the Present: New Studies on Medicine Before, During, and After the Holocaust*, ed. Sabine Hildebrandt, Miriam Offer and Michael A. Grodin (Berghahn Books, 2020), 257–75.

67 See Isabelle Von Bueltzingsloewen, 'Starvation in French Asylums during the German Occupation (1940–1945): Methodological Issues in a Comparative Historical Investigation', in *Transnational Psychiatries: Social and Cultural Histories of Psychiatry in Comparative Perspective c.1800–2000*, ed. Waltraud Ernst and Thomas Mueller (Cambridge Scholars Publishing, 2010), 229–43.

68 On the Pavlov versus Freud characterisation (mostly accurate, but with exceptions) see Mat Savelli and Sarah Marks, 'Introduction', in *Psychiatry in Communist Europe*, ed. Mat Savelli and Sarah Marks (Palgrave, 2015), 7–9. For Pavlov's position within the Soviet regime, see Daniel P. Todes, *Ivan Pavlov: A Russian Life in Science* (Oxford University Press, 2014).

69 For discussion of these themes see Grégory Dufaud and Lara Rzesnitzek, 'Soviet Psychiatry Through the Prism of Circulation: The Case of Outpatient Psychiatry in the Interwar Period', *Kritika* 17, no. 4 (2016), 781–803 and Irina Sirotkina and Marina Kokorina, 'The Dialectics of Labour in a Psychiatric Ward: Work Therapy in the Kaschenko Hospital', in *Psychiatry in Communist Europe*, ed. Mat Savelli and Sarah Marks (Palgrave Macmillan, 2015), 27–49. For a counter-example, in which the nervous disorder neurasthenia, understood in the nineteenth century as a response to a stressful environment, was 'somaticised' and thus individualised during this period, see Anastasia Beliaeva, 'Creating the New Soviet Man: The Case of Neurasthenia', *Social History of Medicine* 35, no. 5 (2022): 927–45.

70 For an example of the rehabilitation and also disciplining of children during this period see Maria Cristina Galmarini-Kabala, 'Psychiatry, Violence, and the Soviet Project of Transformation: A Micro-History of the Perm Psycho-Neurological School-Sanatorium', *Slavic Review* 77, no. 2 (2018): 307–32.

71 Dufaud and Rzesnitzek, 'Soviet Psychiatry through the Prism of Circulation', 784.

72 Dufaud and Rzesnitzek, 'Soviet Psychiatry through the Prism of Circulation', 784 and 794.

73 Dufaud and Rzesnitzek, 'Soviet Psychiatry through the Prism of Circulation', 800–02; see also Benjamin Zajixek, 'Scientific Psychiatry in Stalin's Soviet Union: The Politics of Modern Medicine and the Struggle to Define 'Pavlovian' Psychiatry, 1939–1953' (PhD thesis, University of Chicago, 2009), 3–6, which includes details of arrests and at least one execution of a psychiatrist deemed a deviationist.

74 On Russian psychoanalysis in the years after the Revolution see Hannah Proctor, '"A Country Beyond the Pleasure Principle": Alexander Luria, Death Drive and Dialectic in Soviet Russia, 1917–1930', *Psychoanalysis & History* 18, no. 2 (2016): 155–82 and Alberto Angelini, 'History of the Unconscious in Soviet Russia: From Its Origins to the Fall of the Soviet Union', *International Journal of Psychoanalysis* 89 (2008): 369–88.

75 For biographical details see John Launer, 'Introduction', in *The Essential Writings of Sabina Spielrein*, trans. and ed. Ruth I. Cape and Raymond Burt (Routledge, 2018), 1–13.

76 See Benjamin Zajicek, 'The Psychopharmacological Revolution in the USSR: Schizophrenia Treatment and the Thaw in Soviet Psychiatry, 1954–64', *Medical History* 63, no. 3 (2019): 249–69.

77 For an example of contemporaneous commentary see Harold Merksey and Bronislava Shafran, 'Political Hazards in the Diagnosis of "Sluggish Schizophrenia"', *British Journal of Psychiatry* 148 (1986): 247–56; for background see Benjamin Zajicek, et al., 'Soviet Psychiatry and the Origins of the Sluggish Schizophrenia Concept, 1912–1936', *History of the Human Sciences* 31, no. 2 (2018): 88–105.

78 On the use of psychiatry to persecute dissidents, see Anastassiya Schacht, 'Power in Psychiatry: Soviet Peer and Lay Hierarchies in the Context of Political Abuse of Psychiatry', *History of Psychiatry* 33, no. 1 (2022): 21–33 and Rebecca Reich, *State of Madness: Psychiatry, Literature, and Dissent after Stalin* (Northern Illinois University Press, 2018).

79 See Marks and Savelli, 'Introduction', 13–19. On Yugoslavia see Ana Antic, *Non-aligned Psychiatry in the Cold War: Revolution, Emancipation and Reimagining the Human Psyche* (Palgrave, 2021).

80 For an overview see Mariano Plotkin, 'Freud and the Latin Americans: A Forgotten Relationship', in *Psychoanalysis in the Barrios: Race, Class, and the Unconscious*, ed. Patricia Gherovici and Christopher Christian (Routledge, 2018), 21–37.

81 See Mariano Ben Plotkin, 'Freudian Slips: On the Complicated—and Lingering—Legacy of Psychoanalysis in Argentina', *World Policy Journal* 35, no. 1 (2018): 16–22.
82 See Alejandro A. Dagfal, 'Psychology and Psychoanalysis in Argentina: Politics, French Thought, and the University Connection, 1955–1976', *History of Psychology* 21 (2018): 254–72.
83 G.P. Korman, N. Viotti, and C.J. Garay, 'The Origins and Professionalisation of Cognitive Psychotherapy in Argentina', *History of Psychology* 18, no. 2 (2015): 205–14; on the dissident analysts see Nancy Caro Hollander, 'Psychoanalysts Bearing Witness: Trauma and Memory in Latin America', in *Psychoanalysis in the Barrios*, ed. Gherovici and Christian, 42–43.
84 Dagfal, 'Psychology and Psychoanalysis in Argentina', 266.
85 Plotkin, 'Freudian Slips', 18.

4

UNIVERSALS

In the decades after the Second World War, psychopharmaceuticals and associated shifts in psychiatric knowledge and the legacies of wartime brought biomedical and epidemiological concepts to the field of mental health. Whereas the previous chapter traced these developments at the level of the nation state, in this chapter I consider the impact of this always-transforming psychiatric knowledge in colonial and transnational contexts—in particular, the way psychiatry and mental health were mobilised in the service of colonial psychiatry, as well as the more idealistic and self-consciously global post-war project of producing emotionally stable 'world citizens.' As I will suggest, whether Anglo-European psychiatric knowledge was imposed via colonial rule, proffered via the new forms of international health governance that arose after the Second World War or, more recently, administered via humanitarian aid programs as part of the 'Movement for Global Mental Health' (MGMH), practitioners were repeatedly confronted—and confounded—by the same fundamental question: whether psychiatric illnesses ought to be understood as universal conditions expressed with minor variations across all human societies, or whether forms of mental distress were better characterised as unique to the culture (or, for some clinicians, the racial group) to which the patient belonged. As with the use of psychiatric knowledge for and against the state across the course of the twentieth century, what we might designate as the universalist and the anti-universalist positions were available to actors across the political spectrum, and were deployed to make cases for and against colonialism, international governance, and globalisation. The history of these debates gives some context to the ongoing controversies regarding the alleged neo-imperialism of MGMH and the field of global health more broadly.

DOI: 10.4324/9780429351464-5

Colonial psychiatry

A precursor to the post-war governance of mental health was the field of colonial psychiatry, a term that encompasses both a corpus of racialised theory on the psychic status of colonial subjects and the actual practice of psychiatry in colonial contexts—most visibly, via the spread of colonial asylums.[1] As with the broader imperial health regimes in which it was enclosed, colonial psychiatry reinforced colonial power by supplanting local traditions, hierarchising institutional care via racial categories, and—in keeping with psychiatry's broader propensity to see pathology in purported inferiors—by offering up 'natives' to the scrutiny of white medicine. Colonial psychiatry also policed and reinforced the borders of whiteness and other social categories, in colonial territories and settler states alike. Indeed, the colonial administrators who suffered from 'tropical neurasthenia' and other maladies disclosed a central paradox of 'enlightened' imperialism: that Europeans of dubious heredity might well inflict their own pathologies on those they proposed to uplift.[2]

In addition to these general trends, the theory and practice of colonial psychiatry also reflected the local instantiations of imperial power. In French North Africa, clinicians pursued a program of radical therapeutic reform allied to a biological ethnopsychiatry in which Muslim patients were characterised as innately childish and aggressive. But in French Indochina, by comparison, ideas about psychopathology and its treatment were negotiated through a complex interchange between colonial authorities and the Vietnamese public.[3] In East and Central Africa, British colonial psychiatry was not so much interested in distinguishing 'sane' from 'insane' Africans as in demonstrating the collective inferiority of the African mind.[4] Yet this weight of local circumstance is one indication that the daily exercise of colonial authority could be contingent and fragmentary, even as its cumulative effects were brutal and totalising. Historians' close attention to the influence of local conditions and local actors suggests that, alongside its utility as a technique of rule, colonial health and medicine was, like many other aspects of imperial ventures, often 'hybridized, pluralist, nuanced, and complex.'[5]

There are many instances of such exchanges in the field of psychiatry. In India, for example, long traditions of religious and medical syncretism produced a multivalent concept of madness to which European theorists were latecomers.[6] Similarly, scholarship on the reception of Anglo-European psychiatry in contexts as disparate as Lebanon and Fiji suggests a constant process of (re)negotiation in which imperial, missionary, and local actors shaped ideas about the meanings of madness and the care of the insane.[7] A parallel tendency is evident beyond hospital walls—for example, in the reception of psychoanalysis in the Islamic world and in India.[8] Like psychiatry more broadly, psychoanalysis could operate both as a 'colonial discipline' and as an anti-colonialist critique—as we will see, a double tendency laid bare in the decades after the Second World War.[9] A similar dynamic is evident in the broader field of colonial medicine, where the *absence* of colonial medical personnel, resources, and infrastructure mattered as much as heavy-handed intervention, galvanising anti-colonial sentiment and supplying grounds for a 'critique of colonial neglect' amplified by increased international scrutiny.[10] As Hans Pols has shown, health concerns in the Dutch East Indies, including the 'high prevalence of disease among the indigenous population,' provided nationalists with 'methods, styles of thinking, and biological and physiological metaphors, for evaluating colonial society and diagnosing its ills.'[11] In India, too, Western-trained Indian physicians criticised colonial administrators for their lack of interest and investment in medical infrastructure.[12]

During the period of decolonisation, however, the stakes were clearer. Psychiatric formulations could be used to discredit anti-colonial movements by positioning emergent nationalism as a species of psychopathology, an interpretation that reflected the operational (rather than simply therapeutic) bent of Cold War military psychiatry.[13] British counterinsurgency strategy in Malaya (1948–1960) and Kenya (1952–1960), for example, marshalled psychologised terms such as 're-education' and 'rehabilitation' to justify the extended imprisonment of insurgents in detention camps.[14] In Malaya in the early 1950s, officials keen to better understand captured Chinese Malayan rebels administered questionnaires to ascertain the psychology that underlay their political commitments.[15] In Kenya, colonial authorities were particularly invested in casting the Mau Mau rebellion and the Kikuyu fighters as products of atavistic religious mania—an interpretation advanced by the writings of self-styled experts like the archaeologist Louis Leakey and the psychiatrist J.C. Carothers. Though viewed sceptically by the scholarly community, these interventions nevertheless contributed to a view of the rebels as disordered.[16]

Proponents of such theories could also elide their racial underpinnings. Carothers, for example, proposed that rather than being biologically innate, African inferiority was due to culture and environment and their effects on 'total personality development,' rather than a lack of an essential intelligence. As he argued in a 1951 article in the *Journal of Mental Science*, Africans were conceptually very similar to 'European psychopaths,' so that there was a 'striking resemblance between African thinking and that of leucotomized Europeans.'[17] (Here there were echoes of Freud's equivalence between 'savages and neurotics' in *Totem and Taboo* (1913), as well as his broader if more surreptitious instantiations of recapitulation theory applied to the psyche.[18]) The African 'uses his frontal lobes very little,' Carothers explained, and these 'idle' frontal lobes explained the African's habitual 'unreliability.'[19] Recounting a series of 'failures' by African employees (described in the article as 'domestic servants, mental health attendants, laboratory employees'—workers clearly in the service of Carothers, his wife, and his friends), Carothers appeared conveniently oblivious to the underlying dynamics of the colonial situation. To take a characteristic example, Carothers offered the following scenario, probably furnished by his wife, as evidence of what he dubbed an African employee's 'unreasoning following of a routine':

> The egg-boy brings eggs on Mondays and Thursdays. He failed to come last Thursday on account of the rain, so he did not come again till Monday, though there was nothing to prevent his coming on Friday.[20]

In other words, it was rational to *deviate* from an established routine if it served the needs of the white employer. As the American psychiatrist Kenneth Colby reported acerbically in *Psychoanalytic Quarterly*, Carothers' article offered 'one of the more complete guides to the lowest levels of psychiatric thinking and writing, an example of psychiatry in the service of class prejudice.'[21] Carothers repeated a somewhat attenuated version of his theories in *The Psychology of Mau Mau*, published in 1955. Here, he underplayed the notion that there were 'intrinsic' differences between the minds of Europeans and those of Africans, writing instead that 'in general it can be said that the minds of men (unlike their bodies) are mainly productions of their cultures.'[22] He also conceded that the appeal of Mau Mau, as against loyalty to Britain, was a matter of not just religion but politics:

> Rightly or wrongly, a Kikuyu believes that his political status will not depend in Kenya solely on his merits as a man. In these circumstances, loyalty in the full sense of the word is hardly to be looked for at the moment.[23]

Of course, for colonial authorities, these pathologies were no less real just because they were cultural; if anything, such interpretations offered a means to break anti-colonial resistance by disrupting cultural life, a logic that justified measures like 'villagisation' and detention camps.[24] In the camps, too, physical punishments existed alongside a rhetoric of 'rehabilitation' that attempted to render imprisonment both a punitive and a therapeutic undertaking through which detainees were 'cured' of their extremism.[25] British officials were particularly confounded by the important role played by women in supplying and supporting the rebels. 'Re-education' could thus have a gendered element. In the detention camp at Kamiti, 'hardcore' women were to be rehabilitated via a work and education program emphasising domestic labour.[26] Formal psychiatric treatment was even mooted for the most recalcitrant, though this plan was abandoned due to officials' concerns about the potential fallout of using ECT on female detainees (a telling commentary on the complex perceptions of this treatment).[27]

Yet it was also possible to turn these psychiatric precepts against the coloniser. This played out in French North Africa during the Algerian War of Independence (1954–1962), where the paradoxes of French colonial psychiatry—'modernising while racialising, reforming while conservative'—were parlayed into a catalysing critique of colonialism by the young Martinique-born, French-trained psychiatrist Frantz Fanon.[28] While Fanon arrived in Algiers as an instrument of colonial medicine, he left as a revolutionary, issuing dire warnings about the inevitability (and, he thought, necessity) of decolonial violence, insofar as he regarded colonialism as 'violence in its natural state,' which would 'only yield when confronted with greater violence.'[29] When he joined the sprawling Blida-Joinville hospital in Northern Algeria at the end of 1953, the 'Algiers School' had an enviable reputation for therapeutic innovation, fostered by the hospital's energetic founder Antoine Porot. While much of this work was concerned with elaborating the effectiveness of the new somatic therapies developed in the interwar period—ECT and psychosurgery were liberally prescribed for the hospital's patients—a parallel program of work put a new and putatively scientific gloss on an older theme: the inferiority of the North African mind. Porot and others argued that this was both biologically constituted and reinforced by Muslim 'primitivism' and that it surfaced in the mixture of lassitude and aggression displayed by (male) North African patients—a more 'savage' form of madness than that afflicting the European patients, who resided in separate wards in the segregated hospital. This biological ethnopsychiatry not only naturalised French settler rule outside the hospital walls but conceptualised North African nationalist violence as pathological and inchoate.[30] As was the case with Kenya under the British, anti-colonial unrest was conceived as psychopathological rather than political.

To Fanon, however, this separation between politics and psychic life was a fiction, for he understood all too well the psychic costs of complicity with a colonial regime. His childhood in French-controlled Martinique; his medical training in Lyon, where he treated the city's North African immigrants; his residency at the Saint-Alban hospital under the radical psychiatrist François Tosquelles; and his own experience of racial alterity as a Black man living in France all confirmed the fundamental irreconcilability of the colonial situation.[31] In this respect, the hospital at Blida-Joinville was a microcosm of political life, an institution reproducing colonial hierarchies. Thus, during his 3 years at Blida-Joinville he would insist that in addition to its other depredations, colonialism was also a psychological condition, one that afflicted the coloniser as well as the colonised. Rather than interpret his Arab patients' symptoms as evidence of constitutional abnormality, Fanon emphasised the importance of the political situation in creating psychological distress; if these patients displayed passivity, suspicion and sublimated aggression in clinical settings, it was because they lived in a state of pervading tension. As he put it in his resignation letter of December 1956, '[m] adness is one of the ways that humans have of losing their freedom. And I can say that, placed at this junction, I have measured with terror the extent of the alienation of this country's inhabitants.'[32]

By this point, escalating violence between the French government and the Algerian National Liberation Front (FLN) had made Fanon's position increasingly untenable. After his resignation from Blida-Joinville, he was promptly expelled from Algeria; in time, he landed in Tunisia, where he edited *El Moudjahid*, the newspaper of the FLN, established and ran a psychiatric outpatient clinic at the Hôpital Charles-Nicolle in Tunis, and acted as a roving FLN envoy.[33] In 1961, he died of leukaemia, aged just 36. If he is now best remembered for his most polemical and controversial writings on the necessity of anti-colonial violence, it also bears emphasising that in the last phase of his career he was also practising a kind of anti-colonial, nationalist psychiatry in the outpatient clinic in Tunis. Elsewhere in Africa decolonisation also prompted hopes for the development of new 'national' forms of psychiatry, as well as distinctively African responses to mental distress. That the attempt to realise these aspirations replicated old tensions between the universal and the particular, and that old forms of colonial domination would prove amenable to reproduction by practices of international health governance, speaks to the ongoing struggle to decolonise the (putatively) post-colonial.[34]

World citizens

The psychologised elements of decolonisation in Africa and Asia were complemented (and complicated) by the emergence of international health governance in the decades after the Second World War. In addition to their claims of underwriting geopolitical stability, the United Nations (UN), the World Health Organization (WHO), and associated bodies such as the United Nations Educational, Scientific and Cultural Organization (UNESCO) positioned international health aid as a means to jettison dependent colonial relationships and forge a path towards self-government. The complexities of this aspiration—the capacity of these international organisations to both help nationalist ambitions and sustain colonial hierarchies—have been well-documented, not least because bodies such as the WHO and UNESCO were dominated by Anglo-American personnel (including J.C. Carothers, who published a book-length treatment of 'the African mind' under the WHO's imprimatur).[35] Yet when it came to psychiatry and allied disciplines, there was a bigger agenda still: the articulation of a 'global psyche' as the basis for world citizenship.

The wartime context is key here. In the Anglo-American sphere, psychiatry had demonstrated its utility during the Second World War, and in the tense atmosphere of the early Cold War, it was hoped that psychological knowledge might be similarly mobilised to promote global harmony. There were two tranches to this 'global utopian psychiatry.'[36] The first was technocratic: an initiative, as Harry Wu's work has shown, to establish a standard of 'universal psychopathology' and thus formulate a universal classification system for psychiatric disorders. This initiative reflected post-war efforts in other medical and scientific fields to produce standardised terminology and procedures, as well as clinicians' perennial frustration with the imprecision of psychiatric language.[37] The second group of initiatives was more encompassing and ambitious: to promote the widespread attainment of good mental health as the path to collective emotional stability, 'world citizenship' and world peace. As we will see, bound up with this effort was the pursuit of a transcultural psychiatry—a worldview ostensibly separate from the racialised ethnopsychiatry of colonialism, but in practice containing its own assumptions and blind spots.[38]

There were precedents for these international health measures dating from before the Second World War, mostly to do with the control of diseases such as cholera and plague in the context of increasing international mobility from the mid-nineteenth century onwards. The rationalisation of quarantine measures, via mechanisms such as the 1903 International Sanitary Conference and the establishment of the International Office of Public Hygiene in 1907, offers one example.[39] In terms of mental health, however, it was the mental hygiene movement that forged strong international networks during this period. In 1919, Clifford Beers founded the International Committee for Mental Health (ICMH) to spread the message of prevention; by the time the ICMH held its first International Congress in Washington DC in 1930, it attracted thousands of delegates from over 20 countries.[40] Influential private organisations also interceded. The Rockefeller Foundation was also important for funding international health research, including research into psychiatry and mental health, during the interwar period. Its International Health Commission (later the International Health Division) funded work on infectious diseases, such as hookworm, yellow fever, tuberculosis, and malaria, as well as research fellowships for the study of mental health.[41]

These precursors established precedents around both surveillance and cooperation, to which the six destructive years of the Second World War gave further impetus. The momentum of wartime psychiatric work, which had been concerned with the expeditious treatment of large numbers of casualties, found ongoing expression in these post-war circumstances. But it was hardly an ecumenical effort. The most vocal proponents were American and British clinicians, who brought their assumptions about what constituted a healthy and productive individual; how much they conceived of this work in a truly international frame (as applicable to the war-damaged populations of Asia, for example) is unclear.[42] Finally, in the context of the early Cold War, concern for mental health and health aid itself had an unavoidably geopolitical element. After all, what were presented as international goals were still administered via the unit of the nation state, and reconstruction in Europe was at its core a political exercise. For Western democracies, the creation of healthy and prosperous communities was a bulwark against the lure of political extremism. The United States poured money into devastated parts of Europe where populations suffered from malnutrition and various communicable diseases to blunt incipient communist sympathies. The Soviet Union pursued an analogous aid program in Eastern Europe and the Third World.[43]

Post-war international governance reflected these aims. Promoting health was a central mandate of the United Nations, evidenced by the early creation of the WHO. Its constitution was signed in June 1946, and its formal program began in April 1948; a Mental Health Unit was established in the WHO headquarters in 1949.[44] Its initial concerns were the predictable and pressing ones: standardising nomenclature and advancing programs to combat malaria and smallpox. But its overall agenda was wider than this, because 'health' was conceived very broadly, as a 'state of complete physical, mental and social well-being' and 'not merely the absence of disease or infirmity.' Achieving this measure of health was 'one of the fundamental rights of every human being.' Mental health was thus part of the WHO's program from the outset under its first Director General, the Canadian psychiatrist George Brock Chisholm. He was explicit that psychological states influenced war and politics. As he argued in a speech to the American Psychological Association in September 1948 (later printed in *Science*):

> The uncomfortable fact is that very few people indeed can love themselves in a healthy natural way which tolerantly accepts all their own human urges as normal and inevitable aspects of the healthily functioning man or woman. . . . The anxiety engendered motivates the projection of these feelings of despising, distrust, and hate on to other people. . . . The consequent aggressive feelings against such people are experienced as virtuous. It appears that a system which imposes an early belief in one's own sinfulness, or unacceptability in one's natural state, with its consequent inferiority feelings and anxiety, must be harmful to interhuman relationships and to the ability of the human race to survive in the kind of world this has become.

In order to achieve the kind of 'world citizenship' that Chisholm and other post-war internationalists envisaged, the world needed 'large numbers of people in every country who have grown emotionally beyond national boundaries and are sufficiently mature to be capable of being "world citizens".' In other words, international harmony required a kind of psychological equilibrium—a 'maturity' that allowed people to look beyond their own narrow national interests. 'Very few such people have been developed,' argued Chisholm, 'but it is clear that they are the prototype of what the world must have, in large numbers, before there can be any reasonable degree of assurances that the human race will survive for even another generation.'[45] Here, the legacy of the Second World War and the atomic anxiety of the early Cold War is evident, as well as the universalist prescriptions of the WHO's post-war vision, in which political structures were imagined in the form of Western liberal democracies. Wartime changes to psychiatry's professional identity were also relevant (changes that, not coincidentally, reinforced psychiatry's usefulness in the post-war era). As a 1962 WHO report on its mental health work put it, the war had created 'a new kind of psychiatrist,' one 'engaged largely in preventative work away from the institutional atmosphere,' who had 'many opportunities for operational research' and who could perform such useful post-war work as 'fitting men into jobs for which they were mentally and temperamentally suitable.'[46] This now extended to the international sphere, where psychiatric knowledge could be used to form new international subjects.

The WHO's aspirations for mental health were carried forward by two subsidiary bodies established at the International Congress of Mental Health, held in August 1948. Delegates to this meeting came from several disciplinary backgrounds, indicating the degree disciplines such as sociology and anthropology had been first psychologised during the interwar period and then instrumentalised during the war itself. The World Federation of Mental Health (WFMH—formerly the International Committee for Mental Hygiene) was led by the British psychiatrist J.R. Rees and featured Chisholm, Harry Stack Sullivan, and Margaret Mead as prominent members—all individuals whose wartime experiences caused them to regard mental health and world peace as closely related.[47] The WFMH's first publication, *Mental Health and World Citizenship* (1948), proposed that the 'ultimate goal' of the mental health movement was to enable people to live peaceably with one another and positioned the family as the key determinant of psychosocial adjustment.[48] In contrast, the concerns of the Expert Committee on Mental Health were more technical and related to the 'incorporation into public-health work of the responsibility for promoting the mental as well as the physical health of the community,' the importance of prevention and the reform of institutions in both the developed and the developing world—in particular, the replacement of the old custodial asylum with a 'comprehensive mental health service' that intervened before the patient required protracted hospitalisation. At the same time, uncertainties about Western psychiatric institutions interceded: a later report conceded that 'the psychiatric hospital of European or North American pattern might prove less suitable for Asia than some form of community care' and that Western child guidance programs 'might need to be modified' to be useful to children in non-Western contexts.[49]

These efforts dovetailed with increased attention to the way psychiatric disorders were described and classified—a problem that clinicians had been trying to solve since the nosological investigations of Emil Kraepelin in the late nineteenth century (and which had also prompted Kraepelin's epidemiological inquiries in Java.)[50] Standardised nomenclature was both fundamental to the project of universal psychiatry and frustratingly elusive, as the histories of the *International Statistical Classification of Diseases and Related Health Problems* (ICD) and the American Psychiatric Association's *Diagnostic and Statistical Manual* (DSM) show.[51] In the international sphere, the challenge lay not just in reconciling various competing 'psy' paradigms, but in accounting for the influence of a patient's culture and environment. Whereas colonial psychiatry had tended to racialise patients' symptoms and suggest that colonial subjects suffered from distinct and inferior forms of madness, proponents of post-war international psychiatry saw universal conditions mediated through culture—although, as we have seen in the case of Carothers, 'culture' could be instrumentalised by ethnopsychiatry as well. An added complication was the fact that some 'colonised' clinicians *also* endorsed the existence of distinctive ethnic psychopathologies as part of a wider ethnonationalist agenda.[52]

For the universalists, psychiatric epidemiology and its application to the study of schizophrenia was an important avenue for expounding this worldview. In 1966, an International Pilot Study of Schizophrenia (IPSS), conducted under the auspices of the WHO and drawing on the expertise of the Taiwanese psychiatrist and epidemiologist Tsung-Li Lin, appeared to establish both that schizophrenia was a universal disorder but also that patient outcomes were strongly influenced by the local environment and prevailing culture.[53] Most notably, on certain measures of recovery ('complete clinical remission,' 'longer periods of community functioning,' less continuous anti-psychotic medication), patients in Nigeria, India, and Colombia appeared to do better than patients in the United States, Britain, the USSR, and Denmark, probably because, in a reflection of Wing and Brown's work on institutionalism, they were not so readily hospitalised.[54]

While the IPSS was 'a milestone in the post-war search for universal dimensions of human psychology,' traces of the old ethnopsychiatry—such as the use of evolutionary paradigms to explain (and implicitly hierarchise) the expression of emotion in different cultures—remained.[55] In this sense, the IPSS reflected an underlying epistemological tension in the new field of transcultural psychiatry, a strand of theory formally inaugurated by researchers at McGill University in the 1950s, though still temperamentally linked to the WHO's wider project. Advocates of transcultural approaches argued that the kind of universalism being propounded by the WHO was conceived in entirely Western terms, in effect denying the existence of so-called 'culture-bound' syndromes.[56] In their pioneering studies into schizophrenia and depression across several national contexts, the McGill researchers proposed that culture had a powerful determining role in the way symptoms were expressed.[57] Reporting on the depression study, for example, the researchers concluded that while national cultures did not influence the frequency of psychotic depression per se, 'the level of cohesion in the community and hence the degree to which the individual feels himself involved in social expectations' did. Cultures also shaped the kinds of symptoms patients experienced: for example, in one study, 'intensity of religious involvement' in Judaeo-Christian contexts appeared to be associated with 'a form of depression in which guilt and self-depreciation loom large.'[58] Yet at the same time, early issues of *Transcultural Psychiatry* suggest a parallel interest in documenting 'culture bound' syndromes rather than universalising them.[59] The lines between culture and biology were not clear.

In this regard, growing dissatisfaction with transcultural psychiatry was perhaps inevitable. In 1977, an influential article by the American psychiatrist and anthropologist Arthur Kleinman proposed the adoption of a 'new cross-cultural psychiatry.' The problem with transcultural psychiatry, he argued, was that it had used epidemiology to validate the universality of disease categories that were themselves Western conceits, and this had resulted in a corresponding conflation of 'disease' and 'illness' that elided the nuances of both concepts. Kleinman argued for an anthropological sensibility that appreciated the way culture shaped the perception and experience of disease and illness without the overlay of Western categories.[60] Yet disagreement about how best to incorporate the influence of different cultural contexts continued. Writing in 1990, Roland Littlewood (another psychiatrist and anthropologist) argued that the problem was deeper and more thoroughgoing than the proponents of either transcultural or cross-cultural psychiatry allowed. The fact was that not only did psychiatry have 'no rigorous theory for dealing with the dialectical interplay of biology and human society,' but it also had no template for 'examining the relationship between psychopathologies and its own procedures of research and practice.'[61] As such, the tension between the universal and the particular in cross-cultural contexts is nested in the ongoing negotiation between biology and culture, which globalisation only attenuates.[62]

Global mental health

If the WHO's championing of a universal psyche was a response to the devastation of the Second World War, the advent of global mental health (GMH) as a mainstay of international governance was prefigured by a reorientation away from idealism and towards pragmatism. Beginning in the 1970s, the WHO began to turn its attention to 'standard making and enforcement of norms'—a policy-first orientation that foreshadowed a neoliberalist turn in international health and aid governance that has generated a large amount of critical commentary.[63] At the same time, renewed international interest in human rights violations during this period, and the visibility of the anti-psychiatry movement, underscored the potential for authoritarian regimes to use psychiatry against opponents, as well as the capacity of commonplace psychiatric measures to violate the rights of individual patients. While the animating sentiments may have been laudable, critics charge that the focus on individual rights came at the expense of attention to more entrenched structural issues such as the adequacy of health funding, and that this focus on the individual also supported an increasingly marketised approach to quantifying both physical and mental health (as well as 'underdevelopment' generally) in economic terms—as lost productivity or economic 'burden.'[64] Critics point out that as well as eliding the experience of actual distress, such metrics may not be entirely rigorous and also do nothing to ameliorate systemic inequalities.[65] For example, though much has been made of the capacity of non-specialists to bridge the treatment gap between the Global South and the Global North—an aspiration that draws, not unproblematically, on existing infrastructure in fields such as global HIV/AIDS treatment and prevention[66]—this also risks reproducing the same inequity it wishes to solve. In that respect, systemic under-resourcing can masquerade as cultural sensitivity—a frustration for many critics of the broader field of 'development' in which piecemeal, individualised measures vastly outweigh genuinely redistributive programs.[67] It can also distract from more pervading causes of mental distress, such as poverty and violence.

Critics have also taken issue with some more clinical elements of global mental health. As international humanitarianism increasingly espoused a therapeutic mission, it attracted accusations of promoting a kind of neo-imperialist psychiatry. Particular attention has been paid to the presence of Western clinicians in disaster zones, using post-traumatic stress disorder (PTSD) to practise what amounted to 'therapeutic imperialism.'[68] The globalisation of psychopharmacology has also attracted similar concern, raising questions about the cultural effects of these drugs, the rapacity of companies in seeking new markets and patients' capacity to consent to these 'modern' treatments when, as one scholar has put it, 'the very mechanism of diagnosis is made in foreign, alien terms.'[69] Yet it would be equally distorting and condescending to deny patients in the Global South access to psychopharmaceuticals on purist political grounds or to valorise 'traditional practices' as always humane, particularly for people suffering from psychoses and other serious psychiatric illnesses.[70]

The practice of 'offshoring' of randomised controlled trials (RCTs) captures this ambivalence. On the one hand, it might be argued that globalising therapeutic RCTs diversifies testing regimes and thus challenges the tendency for medical research to focus on white male bodies, and that it also familiarises patients and clinicians outside the Global North with efficacious and thus potentially lifesaving treatments.[71] Yet insofar as RCTs *necessarily* instrumentalise bodies, and insofar as RCTs conducted in the Global South appear to stem from commercial imperatives first and foremost, this seems an overly optimistic interpretation. Economic disparities (for both test subjects and the clinicians recruited to care for them), underdeveloped medical infrastructure, and imperfect ethics regimes may magnify the risks of exploitation for little ultimate benefit.[72] This then goes to the broader question of how knowledge about mental health is created. Do experts in the Global South get to do research (and publish research, and get credit for research) that informs GMH frameworks, and the project of global health more generally? Some projects are underway.[73] But if they do not, then there is good reason to think that GMH will remain vulnerable to the charge that it is an imperial project.

Conclusion: decolonising mental health

In addition to formal struggles for national liberation, ideas about mental health have found a place in other analogous forms of restitutive politics. The 'liberation psychology' popularised in Latin America and characterised by the work of the murdered priest and psychologist Ignacio Martín-Baró is one example of the way ideas about mental health might be mobilised for political change.[74] Similarly, contemporary Indigenous psychologies offer new possibilities for conceptualising and healing mental distress. If the history of psychiatry and adjacent disciplines shows that Indigenous patients have been misunderstood, marginalised and mistreated by mainstream clinicians, contemporary Indigenous psychologies speak back to settler societies, proposing that the conceptualisation of mental illness as an individualised, medical problem is inadequate: at odds with the collective orientation of Indigenous communities, and insufficiently sensitive to the ongoing effects of dispossession, colonisation, and environmental destruction.[75] Indigenous researchers point to the compounding harms of these 'epistemological tensions' between Western clinical models and Indigenous experiences, the way Indigenous people are not only at risk of being inappropriately medicalised, but also of avoiding clinical care when it is needed.[76]

Reparative gestures may be one way forward. In 2016, the Australian Psychological Society (APS) made a formal apology to Aboriginal and Torres Strait Islander people, acknowledging a problematic history of engagement with Indigenous Australians, including 'silence and lack of advocacy on important policy matters'—notably the removal of Indigenous children from their families, a widespread practice predicated on often-spurious social welfare claims, and still a deterrent for some Indigenous people seeking mental health care.[77] The apology reflected years of advocacy within the APS led by the Australian Indigenous Psychologists Association (AIPA), as well as longer traditions of health activism by Indigenous clinicians, researchers, and community workers seeking to centre Indigenous priorities, including through the Aboriginal Community Controlled Health Organisations established in the 1970s.[78] One facet of redress is practical: the presence of more Indigenous practitioners within the profession, as well as accreditation standards that require non-Indigenous practitioners to demonstrate a minimum level of cultural competency.[79] Others are more conceptual, such as incorporating the notion of social and economic wellbeing (SEWB) into everyday practice. As a 'multidimensional concept' in which mental health is folded into a broader category of health and wellbeing that includes 'connection to land or "country", culture, spirituality, ancestry, family, and community,' some Indigenous researchers regard SEWB as a more accurate description of what constitutes mental health.[80]

The similarities between SEWB and the socio-political critiques of psychiatry discussed in the following chapters suggest that mainstream psychiatry has much to learn from Indigenous worldviews and their understandings of mental health. Yet the settler reflex to instrumentalise, metaphorise, and commodify Indigenous knowledge will present an ongoing challenge.[81] Indeed, conventional mental health paradigms can have ambiguous effects on Indigenous communities living in the shadow of dispossession and genocide. Just as the history of colonial psychiatry demonstrates the potential for repressive regimes to medicalise dissent, concepts like trauma can be at once a means of repair but also, in the colonisers' hands, a vehicle for stigma.

Finally, though its proponents assert a moral, humanitarian impetus for the effort to make mental health 'global,' psychiatry's historical engagement in transnational and globalised spaces suggests that critics of GMH have good cause to warn of its potential to enact another form of epistemic hegemony over the Global South, over and above the local examples of appropriation and repurposing that were also characteristic of the psychiatry practised within the framework of European imperialism, and despite the existence of an anti-colonialist psychiatry. Perhaps the real problem here is the notion of the 'global' itself, insofar as it is a term that tends towards an uncritical universalism, eschewing not just local conditions but the broader structural disparities between the Global North and South. This is one example of a more thoroughgoing tendency to disavow the sociopolitical elements of mental health that the activists discussed in the next chapter sought to address.

Notes

1 Sloan Mahone and Megan Vaughan suggest two main domains: the institutional and the more theoretical and conceptual. See 'Introduction', *Psychiatry and Empire*, ed. Sloan Mahone and Megan Vaughan (Palgrave MacMillan, 2007), 1–16.

2 For accounts of colonial psychiatry and its various applications to 'natives', administrators and settlers see Richard Keller, 'Madness and Colonization: Psychiatry in the British and French Empires, 1800–1962', *Journal of Social History* 35, no. 2 (2001):

295–326; Waltraud Ernst, *Mad Tales from the Raj: Colonial Psychiatry in South Asia, 1800–58* (Anthem Press, 2010); Catharine Coleborne, *Insanity, Identity and Empire: Immigrants and Institutional Confinement in Australia and New Zealand, 1873–1910* (Manchester University Press, 2015); and Warwick Anderson, 'The Trespass Speaks: White Masculinity and Colonial Breakdown', *American Historical Review* 102, no. 5 (1997): 1343–70.

3 See Richard E. Keller, *Colonial Madness in French North Africa* (University of Chicago Press, 2007) and Claire Edington, *Beyond the Asylum: Mental Illness in French Colonial Vietnam* (Cornell University Press, 2019).

4 For an overview see Megan Vaughan, *Curing Their Ills: Colonial Power and African Illness* (Stanford University Press, 1991).

5 Suman Seth, 'Colonial History and Postcolonial Science Studies', *Radical History Review* 127 (2017): 76.

6 See for example Sanjeev Jain, et al., 'Psychiatry in India: Historical Roots, Development as a Discipline and Contemporary Context', in *Mental Health in Asia and the Pacific: Historical and Cultural Perspectives*, ed. Harry Minas and Milton Lewis (Springer, 2017), 39–55.

7 See Jaqueline Leckie, *Colonising Madness: Asylum and Community in Fiji* (University of Hawai'i Press, 2019) and Joelle M. Abi-Rached, *'Asfūriyyeh: A History of Madness, Modernity, and War in the Middle East* (The MIT Press, 2020).

8 See Shruti Kapila, 'The "Godless" Freud and His Indian friends: An Indian Agenda for Psychoanalysis', in *Psychiatry and Empire*, ed. Mahone and Vaughan, 124–52; Omnia El Shakry, *The Arabic Freud: Psychoanalysis and Islam in Modern Egypt* (Princeton University Press, 2017) and the essays in *Unconscious Dominions: Psychoanalysis, Colonial Trauma, and Global Sovereignties*, ed. Warwick Anderson, Deborah Jenson and Richard C. Keller (Duke University Press, 2011).

9 See Ranjana Khanna, *Dark Continents: Psychoanalysis and Colonialism* (Duke University Press, 2003), 6.

10 Sunil S. Amrith, *Decolonising International Health: India and Southeast Asia, 1930–65* (Palgrave, 2006), 11.

11 Hans Pols, *Nurturing Indonesia: Medicine and Decolonisation in the Dutch East Indies* (Cambridge University Press, 2018), 5.

12 Amrith, *Decolonising International Health*, 23–24.

13 Erik Linstrum, *Ruling Minds: Psychology in the British Empire* (Harvard University Press, 2016), 166–67.

14 For a detailed account of the counterinsurgency strategy in Malaya see Karl Hack, *The Malayan Emergency* (Cambridge University Press, 2021); for Kenya see Huw Bennett, *Fighting the Mau Mau: The British Army and Counter-Insurgency in the Kenya Emergency* (Cambridge University Press, 2012).

15 See Linstrum, *Ruling Minds*, 155–56.

16 Linstrum, *Ruling Minds*, 182–83; on Leakey see also Bruce Berman and John Lonsdale, 'Louis Leakey's Mau Mau: A Study in the Politics of Knowledge', *History and Anthropology* 5, no. 2 (1991): 143–204.

17 J.C. Carothers, 'Frontal Lobe Function and the African', *Journal of Mental Science* 97, no. 406 (1951): 12.

18 Jacqueline Rose, 'Freud in the "Tropics"', *History Workshop Journal* 47 (1999): 49–67.

19 Carothers, 'Frontal Lobe Function and the African', 40.

20 Carothers, 'Frontal Lobe Function and the African', 26–27.

21 K.M. Colby, 'Journal of Mental Science. XCVII, 1951: Frontal Lobe Function and the African. J.C. Carothers. Pp. 12–48', *The Psychoanalytic Quarterly* 21 (1952): 594–95.

22 J.C. Carothers, *The Psychology of Mau Mau* (The Government Printer, Nairobi, 1955), 2.

23 Carothers, *Psychology of Mau Mau*, 19–20.

24 On villagisation as part of British counterinsurgency strategies see Huw Bennett, 'The Mau Mau Emergency as Part of the British Army's Post-War Counter-Insurgency Experience', *Defence & Security Analysis* 23 (2007): 143–63.

25 See A.R. Baggally, 'Myths of Mau Mau Expanded: Rehabilitation in Kenya's Detention Camps, 1954–60', *Journal of Eastern African Studies* 5, no. 3 (2011): 553–78 and David Anderson, 'British Abuse and Torture in Kenya's Counter-insurgency, 1952–1960', *Small Wars and Insurgencies* 23, no. 4–5 (2012): 700–19. On the Hanslope Park 'migrated archives' and other colonial archive erasures see Riley Linebaugh, 'Colonial Fragility: British Embarrassment and the So-called "Migrated Archives"', *Journal of Imperial and Commonwealth History* 50, no. 4 (2022): 729–56.

26 Katherine Bruce-Lockhart, '"Unsound" Minds and Broken Bodies: The Detention of "Hardcore" Mau Mau Women at Kamiti and Gitamaya Detention Camps in Kenya, 1954–1960', *Journal of Eastern African Studies* 8, no. 4 (2014): 590–608. Women's involvement in the uprising was also of interest to Carothers, *Psychology of Mau Mau*, 16, 22.

27 Bruce-Lockhart, '"Unsound" Minds and Broken Bodies', 602.

28 See Camille Robcis, *Disalienation: Politics, Philosophy, and Radical Psychiatry in Postwar France* (University of Chicago Press, 2021), 62.

29 Frantz Fanon, *The Wretched of the Earth*, trans. Constance Farrington (Penguin, [1961] 1967), 48, 72–73.

30 See Keller, *Colonial Madness in French North Africa*, particularly 121–60.

31 For these biographical details see Keller, *Colonial Madness in French North Africa*, 163–64; Robcis, *Disalienation*, 51–61.

32 Frantz Fanon, 'Letter to the Resident Minister', December 1956, in *Alienation and Freedom*, ed. Jean Khalfa and Robert J.C. Young, trans. Steven Corcoran (Bloomsbury Academic, 2018), 434.

33 For a detailed account of Fanon's last years, see the final chapter of David Macey, *Frantz Fanon: A Biography* (Picador, 2000), 301–498; on the day clinic see the (unpublished) papers: Frantz Fanon, 'Day Hospitalization in Psychiatry: Value and Limits' (1959) and (with Charles Geronimi), 'Day Hospitalization in Psychiatry: Value and Limits. Part Two: Doctrinal Considerations', in *Alienation and Freedom*, 473–509.

34 On Nigeria see Matthew M. Heaton, *Black Skin, White Coats: Nigerian Psychiatrists, Decolonization, and the Globalization of Psychiatry* (Ohio University Press, 2013). For developments in Uganda see Yolana Pringle, *Psychiatry and Decolonisation in Uganda* (Palgrave, 2019).

35 Linstrum, *Ruling Minds*, 191; J.C. Carothers, *The African Mind in Health and Disease: A Study in Ethnopsychiatry* (World Health Organization, 1953).

36 See Ana Antić, 'Decolonizing Madness? Transcultural Psychiatry, International Order and Birth of a "Global Psyche" in the Aftermath of the Second World War', *Journal of Global History* 17 (2022): 21–22.

37 Harry Wu, *Mad by the Millions* (MIT Press, 2021), 92–93. For an account of the problems of data collection in the WHO European office, see Steve Sturdy, Richard Freeman and Jennifer Smith-Merry, 'Making Knowledge for International Policy: WHO Europe and Mental Health Policy, 1970–2008', *Social History of Medicine* 26, no. 3 (2013): 532–54.

38 See Emmanuel Delille and Ivan Crozier, 'Historicizing Transcultural Psychiatry: People, Epistemic Objects, Networks, and Practices', *History of Psychiatry* 29 (2018): 257–62.

39 According to Alex Chase-Levenson, the Mediterranean quarantine system constituted 'the largest transnational scheme for preventative medicine before the formation of the WHO': *The Yellow Flag: Quarantine and the British Mediterranean World, 1780–1860* (Cambridge University Press, 2020), 21. For a contemporaneous overview on one of these measures, see 'The International Sanitary Conference, Paris, 1903', in *British Medical Journal*, 12 December 1903, 1549–50.

40 See the account in Mathew Thomson, 'Mental Hygiene as an International Movement', in *International Health Organisations and Movements, 1918–1939*, ed. Paul Weindling (Cambridge University Press, 1995), 283–304.
41 On the mental health initiatives see Edgar Jones and Shahina Rahman, 'The Maudsley Hospital and the Rockefeller Foundation: The Impact of Philanthropy on Research and Training', *Journal of the History of Medicine and Allied Science* 64, no. 3 (2008): 273–99. For an overview of the Foundation's health initiatives see John Farley, *To Cast Out Disease: A History of the International Health Division of the Rockefeller Foundation (1913–1951)* (Oxford University Press, 2003).
42 For discussion see *Traumatic Pasts in Asia: History, Psychiatry, and Trauma from the 1930s to the Present*, ed. Mark Micale (Berghahn Books, 2021) and *Routledge Handbook of Trauma in East Asia*, ed. Tina Burrett and Jeff Kingston (Routledge, 2023).
43 See Michael Holm, *The Marshall Plan: A New Deal for Europe* (Routledge, 2017).
44 *WHO and Mental Health, 1949–1961* (World Health Organization, 1962), 6; on the establishment of the WHO generally see Marcos Cueto, Theodore M. Brown and Elizabeth Fee, *The World History Organization: A History* (Cambridge University Press, 2019), 34–61.
45 George Brock Chisholm, 'Social Responsibility', *Science* 109, no. 2820 (1949): 27–43, 29.
46 *WHO and Mental Health*, 4.
47 See Wu, *Mad by the Millions*, 42–43.
48 *Mental Health and World Citizenship: A Statement Prepared for the International Congress on Mental Health* (World Federation for Mental Health, 1948), 30.
49 *WHO and Mental Health*, 5.
50 See Eric J. Engstrom and Ivan Crozier, 'Race, Alcohol and General Paralysis: Emil Kraepelin's Comparative Psychiatry and His Trips to Java (1904) and North American (1925)', *History of Psychiatry* 29 (2018): 263–81. These authors argue that, contrary to some suggestions, Kraepelin was not an originator of comparative psychiatry but, rather, used these trips to bolster his broader universalist aims regarding specific conditions.
51 For the ICD see Wu, *Mad by the Millions*, 1–10 and throughout; for the DSM, see Hannah Drecker, *The Making of DSM-III: A Diagnostic Manual's Conquest of American Psychiatry* (Oxford University Press, 2013).
52 See discussion in Antic, 'Decolonizing Madness?', particularly 25 and 30.
53 On Lin see Wu, *Mad by the Millions*, 101–13; see also Stephen Pincock, 'Tsung-yi Lin: Obituary', *The Lancet* 377, no. 9763 (2011): 376. On the importance of statistics to global health generally see Yi-Tang Lin, *Statistics and the Language of Global Health: Institutions and Experts in China, Taiwan, and the World, 1917–1960* (Cambridge University Press, 2022).
54 See Heaton, *Black Skin, White Coats*, 98: these findings 'suggested that Western psychiatry had something to learn from non-Western cultures and healing regimes.'
55 Antic, 'Decolonizing madness?', 27–29.
56 One such critic was the psychiatrist Pow Meng Yap; see Ivan Crozier and Emmanuel Delille, 'Introduction: Pow Meng Yap and the Culture-bound Syndromes', *History of Psychiatry*, 29 (2018): 363–85.
57 See H.B.M. Murphy, 'A Cross-Cultural Survey of Schizophrenic Symptomatology', *International Journal of Social Psychiatry* 9, no. 4 (1963): 237–49; the depression study is reported in H.B.M. Murphy, et al., 'Crosscultural Inquiry into the Symptomatology of Depression: A Preliminary Report', *Transcultural Psychiatric Research Review and Newsletter* 1 (1964): 5–18.
58 Murphy, et al., 'Crosscultural Inquiry', 17.
59 See for example the second issue of *Transcultural Psychiatric Research Review and Newsletter* 1, no. 2 (1964), which included a precis of 'kitsunetsuki' (possession by foxes) in Japan, as well as overviews of psychosomatic syndromes in Africa and rates of mental illness in Israel.

60 Arthur M. Kleinman, 'Depression, Somatization and the "New Cross-Cultural Psychiatry"', *Social Science & Medicine* 11 (1977): 3–9.
61 Roland Littlewood, 'From Categories to Contexts: A Decade of the "New Cross-Cultural Psychiatry"', *British Journal of Psychiatry* 156 (1990): 308–09.
62 For discussion see Laurence J. Kirmayer, 'Beyond the "New Cross-cultural Psychiatry": Cultural Biology, Discursive Psychology and the Ironies of Globalization', *Transcultural Psychiatry* 43 (2006): 126–44.
63 See Wu, *Mad by the Millions*, 28.
64 For discussion of how these metrics are generated and understood, see Daniel Arias, et al., 'Quantifying the Global Burden of Mental Disorders and Their Economic Value', *eClinicalMedicine* 54 (2022): 101675.
65 See discussion in Lisa Cosgrove, et al., 'A Critical Review of the Lancet Commission on Global Mental Health and Sustainable Development: Time for a Paradigm Change', *Critical Public Health* 30 (2020): 624–31.
66 For the 'valuable inequalities' produced by global health responses to AIDS in Africa see Johanna Tayloe Crane, *Scrambling for Africa: AIDS, Expertise, and the Rise of American Global Health Science* (Cornell University Press, 2013).
67 See Anindya Das and Mohan Rao, 'Universal Mental Health: Re-evaluating the Call for Global Mental Health', *Critical Public Health* 22, no. 4 (2012): 383–89.
68 See Janaka Jayawickrama and Jo Rose, 'Therapeutic Imperialism in Disaster and Conflict-affected Countries', in *The Routledge International Handbook of Critical Mental Health*, ed. Bruce Cohen (Routledge, 2018), 213–23; see also Didier Fassin and Richard Rechtman, *The Empire of Trauma: An Inquiry into the Condition of Victimhood*, trans. Rachel Gomme (Princeton University Press, 2009).
69 China Mills, *Decolonizing Global Mental Health: The Psychiatrization of the Majority World* (Routledge, 2014), 151.
70 See Arthur Kleinman, 'Global Mental Health: A Failure of Humanity', *The Lancet* 374 (2009): 603–04.
71 See for example Lewis R. Roberts, et al., 'Unmet Needs in Oncology Clinical Research and Treatment in Africa: Focus on Ghana', *The Oncologist* 27, no. 9 (2022): 760–67.
72 See Athula Sumathipala and Buddhika Fernando, 'Ethical Issues in Global Mental Health Trials', in *Global Mental Health Trials*, ed. Graham Thornicroft and Vikram Patel (Oxford University Press, 2015), 123–38. See also S.W. Glickman, et al., 'Ethical and Scientific Implications of the Globalisation of Clinical Research', *New England Journal of Medicine* 360 (2009): 816–23 and Adriana Petryna, *When Experiments Travel: Clinical Trials and the Global Search for Human Subjects* (Princeton University Press, 2009). See also S.D. Taylor-Robinson, et al., 'Why Is There a Paucity of Clinical Trials in Africa?', *QJM: An International Journal of Medicine* 114, no. 6 (2021): 357–58.
73 Forms of instrumentalisation still exist, however. For examples of 'reverse' or 'frugal' innovation, see the collection 'Reverse Innovation in Global Health Systems: Learning from Low-income Countries', *Globalization and Health*, ed. Viva Dadwal, Matthew Harris, and Shams Sye: 1744–860–3 (online); for examples of 'ethics dumping' in North—South collaborations, see *Ethics Dumping: Case Studies from North-South Research Collaborations*, ed. Doris Schroeder, Julie Cook, François Hirsch, Solveig Fenet and Vasantha Muthuswamy (Springer Open, 2018).
74 For an overview see Mark Burton and Raquel Guzzo, 'Liberation Psychology: Origins and Development', in *Liberation Psychology: Theory, Method, Practice, and Social Justice*, ed. L. Comas-Díaz and E. Torres Rivera (American Psychological Association, 2020), 17–40; on the work and legacy of the Spanish-born Jesuit priest and social psychologist Ignacio Martín-Baró, who spent his working life in El Salvador and was assassinated by the military in 1989, see Ignacio Martín-Baró, *Writings for a Liberation Psychology*, ed. Adrianne Aron and Shawn Corne (Harvard University Press, 1996).

75 See the overview in Nuria Ciofal, et al., 'Indigenous Community Psychologies, Decolonisation, and Radical Imagination Within Ecologies of Knowledges', *American Journal of Community Psychology* 69, no. 3–4 (2022): 283–93 as well as W. Waitoki, et al., 'Indigenous Psychology in Aotearoa/New Zealand and Australia', in *Global Psychologies: Mental Health and the Global South*, ed. Suman Fernando and Roy Moodley (Palgrave Macmillan, 2018), 163–84, 164, and Ali Ponturo and Meegan Kilcullen, 'A Systematic Review of Evidence-based Psychological Interventions and Aboriginal and Torres Strait Islander People', *Clinical Psychologist* 25, no. 2 (2021): 198–211, 198.

76 The phrase 'epistemological tensions' is from Lisa Wexler, et al., 'Advancing Suicide Prevention Research With Rural American Indian and Alaska Native Populations', *American Journal of Public Health* 105, no. 5 (2014): 891–99. See also Melissa Taitimu, et al., 'Ngā Whakāwhitinga (Standing at the Crossroads): How Māori Understand What Western Psychiatry Calls "Schizophrenia"', *Transcultural Psychiatry* 55, no. 2 (2018): 153–77.

77 See Australian Psychological Society, 'The APS Apology to Aboriginal and Torres Strait Islander People' (Australian Psychological Society, 2017), https://psychology.org.au/community/reconciliation-and-the-aps/aps-apology.

78 On the development of Indigenous health activism, including in the mental health field, see Graham Gee, et al., 'Aboriginal and Torres Strait Islander Social and Emotional Wellbeing', in *Working Together: Aboriginal and Torres Strait Islander Mental Health and Wellbeing Principles and Practice*, ed. Pat Dudgeon, et al. (2nd ed., Commonwealth of Australia, 2014), 55–58. On the work of the AIPA see Yvonne Clark and Tanja Hirvonen, 'Decolonising Australian Psychology: The Influence of Aboriginal Psychologists', in *Decolonial Enactments in Community Psychology*, ed. Shose Kessi, Shahnaaz Suffla and Mohamed Seedat (Springer Nature, 2021), 213–33.

79 See Australian Psychology Accreditation Council, 'Accreditation Standards for Psychology Programs', 1 January 2019.

80 Gee, et al., 'Aboriginal and Torres Strait Islander Social and Emotional Wellbeing', 55.

81 See Eve Tuck and K. Wayne Yang, 'Decolonization Is Not a Metaphor', *Decolonization: Indigeneity, Education & Society* 1 (2012): 1–40.

5

DISCONTENTS

While the anti-psychiatrists like Thomas Szasz and R.D. Laing discussed in Chapter 1 enjoyed a significant following amongst the counterculture, the upheaval of the 1960s and early 1970s brought about a broader reckoning within mainstream psychiatry, most visibly in the United States. Rather than advocate for the wholesale destruction of psychiatry and related ideas about madness and sanity, critics argued instead for an explicit countenancing of the sociopolitical in conceptualising mental illness and mental health. While some of this activity clearly resonated with the sentiments of the anti-psychiatry movement, its ultimate aim was more reformist and, ultimately, more consequential: that mainstream Freudian psychiatry shed some of its more doctrinaire, untested assumptions about the causes of mental distress—a position that, in the attention it gave to scientific methods, ironically ended up bolstering the biological psychiatrists and sidelining the sociopolitical once again. While historians are increasingly exploring similar themes of 'the social' in the psychiatry of the post-war United States and elsewhere and their effects on understandings of mental illnesses and mental health, here my approach emphasises instances of more explicitly political critique.[1] To do so, I examine the debates over homosexuality and race in the American Psychiatric Association, as well as the rise of 'mad' activism that sought to reclaim the patient's voice.

The sexual politics of diagnosis

The well-known campaign to remove homosexuality from the American Psychiatric Association's *Diagnostic and Statistical Manual* (DSM) is just one instance of psychiatry's long entanglement with questions of sex, gender and sexuality. Feminist scholars have long pointed out that for much of its history psychiatry

DOI: 10.4324/9780429351464-6

exhibited a peculiar and often pernicious interest in women's minds and bodies—factors that may explain women's apparent overrepresentation in custodial institutions and in rates of diagnosis.[2] Similarly, scholarship on the feminisation of a diagnosis like 'hysteria' indicates that assumptions about gender can distort both diagnostic practices and the terminology they mobilise.[3] In contemporary contexts, critical literatures on diagnoses such as a premenstrual dysphoric disorder, premenstrual syndrome, and borderline personality disorder frequently use historicist arguments to question the validity of these labels.[4] During the 1960s, however, Freud and psychoanalysis came under particularly sustained attack from second-wave feminists in the United States. This reflected a complicated legacy. Histories of psychoanalysis suggest that early female analysts and analysands played an important role in the growth of the discipline, as well as in the theorisations of female subjectivity and sexuality that, in the context of *fin de siècle* Central Europe, had a radical edge.[5] Yet in the post-war decades, prominent strands of American psychoanalysis and the ego psychology it espoused had promoted a stultifying gender conformity that for women centred around heterosexual marriage and motherhood. The groundless claims of some psychoanalytic popularisers regarding the superiority of vaginal over clitoral orgasms—a position that conveniently designated the penis as the prime vector of sexual pleasure—were the subject of frequent feminist anger and ridicule (as well as intense theoretical debate in psychoanalytic circles). Finally, advocacy around the incidence of incest and sexual violence towards women and children trained feminist anger on Freud for his eschewal of the so-called 'seduction thesis,' among other crimes.[6]

Simultaneously, however, feminist thinkers—liberals like Betty Friedan as well as radicals like Kate Millet and Shulamith Firestone—used psychologised frameworks to describe and condemn female oppression (notably, Millet and Firestone would go on to have their own bruising experiences as psychiatric patients). As ever, psychological language and concepts could both oppress and potentially liberate. Some feminist theorists sought to debunk elements of psychoanalysis in psychoanalytic terms. Here, in the words of one historian, '[t]he logic of psychoanalytic formulations . . . invaded the camp of declared enemies.'[7] 'Consciousness raising' sessions—which foregrounded women's personal experiences and challenges—often incorporated psychological concepts and enlisted sympathetic therapists as discussion leaders. Finally, practical measures reflected a wider agenda to improve women's healthcare, including women's experiences of therapy. Phyllis Chesler and other feminist psychologists rethought what a truly feminist therapy might look like; as we will see, the women's caucus of the radical psychiatrists in the APA advocated for similar change.[8]

In addition to theorisations of women, psychological attitudes towards homosexuality were influenced by an extensive corpus of writings on sexology and sexual science—the important context in which psychoanalysis's confused position on homosexuality was formed and then promulgated in Cold War America.[9] Historians of sexual science have stressed that, taken together, these endeavours were more interdisciplinary, less repressive and less Eurocentric than we might suppose; nevertheless, the collective effect was to exoticise and so pathologise non-heterosexual sexual practices, bodies that did not accord with standard sex binaries and individuals who did not follow 'natural' gender norms.[10] (In addition to psychologised conceptualisations of homosexuality, some of this prefigures the present controversies over trans medicine, in which psychiatry—which once considered 'transgenderism' a distinct disorder—now assumes a 'gatekeeping' role with respect to 'gender dysphoria.'[11])

While in general the (unstable) category of 'homosexuality' and 'the homosexual' became an object of state interest in the late nineteenth century, in the United States the early Cold War period was a particular flashpoint, one that implicated psychiatrists in official surveillance and punishment but also offered avenues for critique that anticipated the activism of the late 1960s and early 1970s.[12] As well as continuing to regulate sexual norms in the armed forces (an extension of their wartime role in the 'pre-selection' programs of the Second World War), psychiatrists also had an important role in new and encompassing legislation targeting 'sexual psychopaths'—a broad category that included child rapists and other violent sex offenders, as well as same-sex couples engaged in consensual sex.[13] This was a kind of juridical turn, in which interwar associations between homosexuality, delinquency, and schizophrenia were amplified above a more positive 'cultured' depiction of homosexuality.[14] Articles published in the *American Journal of Psychiatry* [*AJP*] in the two decades following the Second World War suggest that the profession's participation in this government harassment was accompanied by rumbling unease about the justification for such persecution. Many contributions to the *AJP* urged that the issue be framed clinically, on the grounds that homosexuality was a psychological abnormality over which the individual had little personal control. A group of psychiatrists surveying the military regulations targeting homosexuals said they could not 'help viewing these unfortunate individuals as patients.'[15] One overview of the legal position of homosexuals, published in the *AJP* in 1956, condemned the 'confusion, prudery, and rigid tradition that surround sodomy and related acts,' while also noting that 'homosexuality either cannot be cured or at best entails a long and extremely costly treatment for even minor modifications.'[16] This therapeutic impulse was both sympathetic and stigmatising, saddling homosexual men and women with what the activist Ronald Gold described as 'the damning label of sickness.'[17] Yet, in some contexts, there were significant practical effects. Psychiatric assessment had an important role in softening the punitive impulse of the sexual psychopathy laws. In a set of cases appearing before the Baltimore courts between 1952 and 1954, for example, the court diverted the offender from prison to psychiatric treatment in every instance where a psychiatric assessment was sought. The handful of offenders without a psychiatric assessment went to prison.[18]

Of course, in private clinical settings, the treatment of homosexual patients also had disciplinary aims, even if undertaken 'freely.' The influence of behaviourism in the United States, Britain, Europe, and elsewhere generated 'aversive' techniques in which the predominantly male patients were taught to associate homosexual desire with physical pain via injections of the nausea-producing chemical apomorphine or painful electric shocks.[19] While psychoanalytic psychotherapists eschewed such methods, their own approach was often protracted and expensive and could be damaging in its own way. Moreover, proving success was difficult, especially given the new impetus, discussed in Chapter 2, to think in numbers rather than cases. In this respect, the Kinsey Report was an early and comprehensive shot across the bow, indicating that sexual preference was often fluid and circumstantial.[20] Other evidence began to accumulate. Studies of overprotective mothers, often said to be responsible for effeminacy and homosexuality in men, failed to show a meaningful effect.[21] A study of teenage lesbians found no evidence of a so-called 'reverse Oedipal complex' in these young women.[22] Finally, the long-posited link between homosexuality and paranoid schizophrenia did not materialise in larger cohort studies.[23] As the psychologist Evelyn Hooker suggested,

> from a survey of the literature it seemed highly probable that few clinicians have ever had the opportunity to examine homosexual subjects who neither came for psychological help nor were found in mental hospitals, disciplinary barracks in the Armed Services, or in prison populations.[24]

Combined with the elusiveness of cures, these cracks in the conceptual edifice provided a strong empirical basis for activists to challenge homosexuality's classification as a disorder at all.

The issue culminated in the early 1970s in a series of public confrontations at the APA's annual meetings over the removal of homosexuality from the DSM. Younger psychiatrists were generally supportive, and the biological psychiatrists were agnostic; the holdouts were older psychoanalysts who had trained in the 1930s and 1940s, understood homosexuality as a disorder of psychosexual development, believed that analysis could be an effective treatment in some cases—and stood to lose a portion of their patients if homosexuality was no longer regarded as a mental illness. One example is the psychoanalyst Irving Bieber—a clinician who regarded himself as an ally of his homosexual patients, who reassured them that homosexuality was 'neither evil nor immoral,' and yet who still argued against the removal of homosexuality from the DSM on the grounds that it was an acquired abnormality that caused 'inherent psychological pain.'[25] Another aggrieved analyst was Charles W. Socarides, who felt unfairly demonised by the activists who characterised psychiatry as homophobic. 'Let us bear in mind,' said Socarides, 'that psychiatrists have been in the forefront in helping homosexuals.'[26]

The activist Ronald Gold agreed, at least to an extent. Appearing in the same APA symposium as Bieber and Socarides, he suggested that 'a false adversary situation has been drawn between psychiatry and Gay Liberation.' Many psychiatrists did mean well, he argued, but their formulations had been twisted, put to malign use. In future, there could be a working partnership: 'We can save you the trouble of treating some people, and we can be a helpful adjunct for many of your patients by pointing them along the road to self-esteem.' If a patient genuinely wanted to change their sexual orientation, then psychiatrists ought not to accept this outright but explore the reason the patient wished to change. 'Such people do need help,' Gold wrote. 'But is it their homosexuality that's doing them in? Or is it something that psychiatry has helped create: irrational fear and hatred of homosexuality?'[27] Judd Marmor, a psychoanalyst of the same vintage as Bieber and Socarides but far more sceptical of doctrinal pieties, echoed Gold's arguments:

> Surely the time has come for psychiatry to give up the archaic practice of classifying the millions of men and women who accept or prefer homosexual object choices as being, by virtue of that fact alone, mentally ill. The fact that their alternative life-style happens to be out of favour with current cultural conventions must not be a basis in itself for a diagnosis of psychopathology. It is our task as psychiatrists to be healers of the distressed, not watchdogs of our social mores.[28]

In late 1973, the Board of Trustees voted to remove homosexuality from the DSM and replace it with 'sexual orientation disturbance,' a new disorder that applied only to homosexuals who were distressed by their sexuality (thus leaving the door open for various therapies). But opponents, led by Bieber and Socarides, pressured the Board for a general vote. Fifty-eight per cent voted in favour of removing homosexuality itself from the DSM. Later, in April 1974, the APA published its 'Position Statement on Homosexuality and Civil Rights,' which declared that 'homosexuality per se implies no impairment in judgment, stability, reliability, or general social or vocational capabilities' and that the APA 'deplores all public and private discrimination against homosexuals.'[29] While this was understandably interpreted as a victory for the gay liberation movement, within the APA it was also understood as a successful attack on the psychoanalysts, orchestrated in part by the 'nosological diplomacy' of Robert Spitzer, the soon-to-be-architect of DSM-III.[30]

Race and mental health

In August 1967, researchers from the Lafayette Clinic in Detroit commissioned several hundred interviews with participants and bystanders affected by the civil unrest that had wracked the city in late July.[31] In an article published nearly 2 years later, these investigators were candid about their own motivations as 'psychosocial investigator(s) who wish(ed) to be relevant' in circumstances of political upheaval. One job for such engaged researchers was to 'take the view of the Black revolution to the white community' by emphasising interviewees' 'racial self-consciousness' and aspirations for 'self-government.' The other task was to shine a light on the 'inconsistent and racist attitudes and behaviour of white people,' which the authors sought to achieve by interviewing a battalion of the Michigan National Guard stationed in Detroit during the uprising. Psychiatry 'may be of particular value in understanding these matters,' the authors wrote, 'because its daily work is to translate the irrational into the rational and understandable.'[32] The paper's unabashed sympathies reflected the commitments of lead author Paul Lowinger, one of the founders of a psychiatrists' Radical Caucus established in the late sixties to challenge the APA on what it regarded as the organisation's disingenuously apolitical stance towards the Vietnam War and other pressing issues of the day, including urban violence.[33] Unlike the more militant fringe of the anti-psychiatry movement, many of these clinicians wanted to reform the discipline from within and pressed for more direct acknowledgement of the role of economic inequality, racism, and militarism in causing psychiatric distress. Lowinger and his colleagues' interpretations of the Detroit unrest were wholly in keeping with this agenda and suggest a distinct optimism about the role of clinicians in restructuring American society, despite the fraught history of psychiatry's involvement in questions about race. Since physicians are 'responsible for the health of the community,' argued Lowinger, it followed that they also 'have a healing role in social pathology.'[34]

These clinical interpretations of urban unrest in the 1960s were framed by older and broader debates about the psychological effects of segregation, economic disadvantage and other forms of racial discrimination on the psyches of Black Americans, as well as older racialised categories of psychiatric disorder that had worked to justify slaveholding and would soon find a second life in eugenic reasoning about intelligence and other 'innate' capacities.[35] From the 1940s onwards, psychiatric knowledge had assumed particular importance in quantifying the harms of white supremacy, a strategy vindicated when the Supreme Court cited psychological research on Black children's self-esteem in its decision to overturn school segregation in *Brown v. Board of Education*.[36] Yet there was always dissension, particularly among Black researchers, about the potential for 'pathologism' to feed racist stereotypes, to downplay the effects of structural inequality and to stoke the messiah complexes of their white colleagues.[37] The controversy over the 1965 Moynihan Report, widely interpreted by both liberals and conservatives as portraying Black families in the ghettos of northern cities as both damaged and damaging, reflected this ambiguity.[38] The central conundrum of how to represent the psychological effects of racism without imputing ongoing inferiority was amplified by psychiatry's perennial confusion about the fundamental roots of psychiatric disorders. Competing aetiological models variously stressed the role of inherent biological factors, the influence of early childhood or the impact of the immediate environment (including the stigmatising 'deprivation' theories[39]). Disagreements about causality also reflected wider uncertainty over the empirical basis of other facets of psychiatric practice, such as diagnosis—a state of affairs on unedifying display in this period during the trial of Robert Kennedy's assassin, when psychiatric experts gave contradictory evidence about the defendant's mental status.[40] It was theoretically possible, then, to regard urban 'rioting' as rational and political, as pathological and criminal, as pathological but also political, or some other explicative combination. The suggested remedies were similarly diverse and included community mental health initiatives, increased social spending coupled to an integrationist agenda, as well as the revolutionary structural change (including Black separatism) endorsed by Lowinger and colleagues.[41]

In addition to intimating an underlying conceptual incoherence, competing interpretations of urban violence fed into broader discord about the direction and purpose of psychiatry, including its role in eliding or ignoring racial injustice. This reflected increased advocacy by Black activists and the wider medical profession emphasising the importance of access to healthcare as central to the civil rights agenda.[42] In this regard, the Radical Caucus was but one of several groups of activist clinicians and patients' rights advocates whose frustrations became evident at the APA's annual meetings in 1969 and 1970. In addition to the campaign by gay activists to remove homosexuality from DSM-II, a Women's Caucus committed itself to combating patriarchy within the profession and in clinical practice.[43] By the end of 1969, there were indications that the APA perceived the need to respond to the expectations of its politically engaged membership. In December the Board of Trustees endorsed a 'Position Statement on Alternatives to Violence.' Citing a 'rising tide of violence as an outcome of conflict in modern society' and the growing expectation that the psychiatric profession be able to contribute to 'conflict resolution,' the APA committed to 'a year's special study and self-development through research and scholarly effort' in order to understand the sources of conflict and paths to prevention.[44] Yet not all APA members were convinced that this was territory into which the organisation ought to venture, a position echoed in the simultaneous debates about the APA's official position on the Vietnam War, as we have seen. As one participant in a 1971 symposium on 'The Psychiatrist, the APA, and Social Issues' put it, 'there are rumblings among our membership both that we have become too involved [in social issues] and that we are not involved enough.'[45] Among other factors, political action imperilled the APA's tax exemption.[46] But could it also, as one editorial in the *AJP* wondered, undermine the goals of therapy? While in the traditional therapeutic encounter psychiatry was committed to the 'production of change,' intervention in 'community conflicts' to promote non-violent outcomes was premised on 'social change on behalf of the powerless.' Was this not, the editorial writer argued, 'a contradiction to the role of neutral mediator in a highly polarised and tense situation?'[47] Here the exasperation of the radical psychiatrists becomes clear: insofar as 'community conflicts' referred to unrest in Black urban areas, resistance to fostering 'social change on the behalf of the powerless' was not, in their view, a neutral position.

Black psychiatrists had long been frustrated by such intransigence. Even compared to the underrepresentation of Black doctors in other medical specialities, the number of Black psychiatrists was vanishingly small and the APA had done little to advance the interests of its Black membership or Black psychiatric patients, including those housed in what were still effectively segregated psychiatric facilities in the South.[48] At the 1969 annual meeting, members of the newly formed Black Psychiatrists of America (BPA) presented the APA Board of Trustees with a list of demands, including increased representation on APA committees. The Board agreed to reserve a permanent position for a BPA member and to establish specialised programs within the APA on 'minority issues,' which in coming years resulted in affirmative action initiatives in residency and other training programs.[49] Proponents of such measures argued that increasing the number of Black clinicians was vital for improving mental health services for urban communities and expanding psychiatric knowledge beyond conventional parameters. As one group of recently qualified Black psychiatrists argued in 1970, '[c]lassical psychoanalytic theory teaches us that some forms of mental illness derive from insoluble intrapsychic conflicts,' meaning that '[o]ther contributing factors such as persistent socio-environmental factors are largely ignored or minimised.' This focus on 'white middle class, psychoanalytic values and biases' skewed the discipline towards the concerns of a white middle-class clientele and away from therapeutic work in disadvantaged urban communities.[50]

While these 'persistent socio-environmental factors' figured prominently in Black clinicians' public interpretations of the causes and meaning of the urban uprisings, they were not necessarily antithetical to accounts that emphasised the role of emotional and other 'intrapsychic' conflicts in explaining civic unrest. Rather, clinicians argued that social, economic, and political circumstances both instigated and then mediated emotional expression. Here, the most salient example was anger—an emotion that for Black Americans could be both politically fraught and physically perilous when expressed in public.[51] During the 'heroic period' of the civil rights movement, activists regarded the public sublimation of anger (and the related capacity to weather the anger and outright violence of white crowds and police) as crucial for mollifying liberal opinion and pursuing a politics of respectability. But by the middle sixties, a younger generation of Black activists questioned the value of public equanimity in the face of continued white hostility and state violence.[52] The Black Power movement, whose leaders had read Fanon, thus positioned mounting Black anger as the logical outcome of continued oppression, albeit with potentially revolutionary ends. Mainstream Black clinicians of differing theoretical orientations also portrayed anger in urban communities as a clinically normal response to lives lived under intense pressure. In their book *Black Rage*, psychiatrists William Grier and Price Cobbs argued that Black anger stemmed from the anxiety and paranoia of living in a hostile society, and that these attitudes were 'adaptive devices' that were 'no more pathological than the compulsive manner in which a diver checks his equipment before a dive or a pilot his parachute.'[53] In a review of their book, the social psychologist Kenneth Clark criticised Grier and Cobbs for their reliance on drive theory and their resulting 'preoccupation' with 'ponderous analysis of the dynamics of interracial sexual behaviour.' Perhaps sensitive to the accusations of pathologism levelled at his own work (with his wife Mamie Phipps Clark, he had carried out the famous 'doll studies' on Black preschoolers' self-esteem cited by the Supreme Court in *Brown v. Board of Education*), he regarded this kind of speculation as spurious and entirely divorced from the 'concrete realities of social problems.'[54] Yet elsewhere he had also acknowledged the place of anger in explaining social unrest, noting in his 1965 classic *Dark Ghetto* the 'oddly controlled rage' of the protestors who confronted the police during the 1964 disturbances in Harlem—a 'rage that seemed to say, during those days of social despair, "We have had enough. The only weapon you have is bullets. The only thing you can do is kill us".'[55]

Prominent Black clinicians like Clark, Grier and Cobbs also noted the role of white pathologies in impeding social reform and maintaining racial tensions. Decades earlier, W.E.B. Du Bois had pointed to the 'public and psychological wage' paid to Southern white workers in the form of 'public deference and titles of courtesy' denied to their Black counterparts.[56] In these newer formulations, whiteness offered a similar mix of economic self-interest and psychological consolation. In setting out the alienation of the oppressed, Frantz Fanon had also implied that colonists suffered from reciprocal and grandiose pathologies, in which a belief in the debased nature of the colonised was essential to their self-conception.[57] Clark similarly argued that Black *and* white Americans harboured a 'ghetto inside,' one that caused lower middle-class whites to view their racial status as a talisman for ongoing economic security, and white liberals to proclaim a pure, colour-blind worldview that collapsed into anger and guilt the moment Black demands became inconvenient.[58] (Black psychiatrists also noted this latter tendency at work among white colleagues.[59]) Drawing on postwar studies of antisemitism, the psychoanalytically inclined Grier and Cobbs proposed that white people displaced onto Black people the 'primarily hateful attitudes' that were really directed at 'parents, children, brothers, strangers, the self, or indeed any person about whom contrary feelings are held.' This was amplified by a 'pervasive climate of prejudice,' particularly in the South. As Grier and Cobbs wryly noted, insofar as culture gave context to intrapsychic mechanisms, the white Southerner 'may be a different kind of victim,' primed for racial violence by a social climate that gave tacit assent to its commission. 'One is amazed to find brilliant, cultured men of the world,' wrote Grier and Cobbs, 'whose hatred of Blacks reaches pathological proportions.'[60] Given the tendency of even sympathetic researchers to treat urban communities as vast observational laboratories, turning the psychiatric gaze back onto white people was implicatively restitutive. But it also proposed an important interpretive symmetry, in which acknowledging white irrationality became a corollary of accepting the rationality of Black anger, which, in turn, implied the inseparability of psychic life from politics. From this standpoint, the optimist viewed social reform as a therapeutic intervention. The nihilist, however, saw prejudice as intractable and social reform as expensive window-dressing.

This recent history contextualises contemporary debates about racial disparities in healthcare—glaringly visible during the COVID-19 pandemic—as well as the utility of intergenerational trauma as a vehicle for redressing historic injustices, and the continually resurfacing controversies about 'race' and 'intelligence.'[61] Yet it also reinforces another persistent theme: the way psychiatric concepts might be used to galvanise resistance as well as pathologise dissent. Psychologised interpretations of the era's other protest movements, and the counterculture in general, provide additional examples of this tendency. Here, psychiatric interpretations were split between favourable accounts of the demonstrators as rational dissenters from an unjust status quo and a benign condescension that cast them as children in unthinking rebellion against authority. Drug use amongst the counterculture formed a particular point of interest, as did its ersatz religiosity and its (purported) emphasis on nonviolence.[62] Psychiatric characterisations of New Left activism were more contentious, in particular the intimations of revolutionary violence that had started to collect around its radical fringes. One commentator implied that, for some, activism obscured destructive and even psychotic impulses.[63] Others argued that participants lacked genuine political commitments. Speaking to the APA in May 1969, the Harvard historian H. Stuart Hughes proposed that the movement's aims were 'basically unpolitical,' with no 'revolutionary aim of seizing the means of production or the implements of power and redirecting them for the benefit of the masses.' Instead, 'the goal is psychological,' at bottom a desire 'to see through, to unmask, to strip—literally as well as figuratively—down to total nakedness.' This explained young activists' 'cult of "confrontation" as a quasi-religious act of witness,' as well as their impatience with incrementalism and their intolerance of dissenting views.[64]

Though antagonistic, Hughes' account chimes with several more recent and less ambivalent histories of youth protest and the counterculture that emphasise psychological scrutiny and self-reform as fundamental activities for committed participants. This was especially the case for white middle-class activists who aspired to radicalism but experienced little material deprivation and oppression in their daily lives. For the militants of the New Left such as the Weather Underground, proclaiming solidarity with independence fighters in the Third World and the Black Power movement at home required concomitant displays of authenticity that ranged from certain modes of dress to espousing and planning for revolutionary violence.[65] Psychiatrists also noticed this tendency. A study of one group of activists arrested during the demonstrations at the 1968 Democratic National Convention noted demonstrators striving after 'explicit congruity,' an 'attempt to act overtly as they think and feel.'[66] For sympathetic clinicians, this rigour did not nullify activists' political claims but, rather, underscored the connections between psychological subjectivity and socio-political conditions. Just as urban unrest could be understood as a predictable response to an unjust environment, the behaviour of young activists was the corollary of their outraged witnessing of real events. The ongoing bloodshed in Vietnam was particularly pertinent here, providing a constant riposte to claims of American exceptionalism and moral clarity.

Conclusion: reclaiming madness

As I indicated at the beginning of this chapter, opposition to establishment psychiatry cannot be reduced to the anti-psychiatrists; instead, during the ferment of the 1960s and 1970s, psychiatry came under attack from several directions. Yet it is worth stressing that the voices of clinicians often predominated—a situation that risked sidelining or instrumentalising patients themselves. Was it possible for patients to speak back to psychiatry authority and, if so, what form might that take? If, as one historian has argued, 'evidence of collective and sustained action among patients' is limited before the twentieth century—either because it did not occur, or because the sources are characteristically constrained—then examples accumulate quickly from the interwar period onwards.[67] Clifford Beers' mental hygiene movement is one early example, though as we have seen, it was soon dominated by clinicians. Then, there are less prominent examples. As we saw in Chapter 1, mid-century research into the social life of asylums and the broader pursuit of therapeutic communities suggested that patients might offer important and often more penetrating insight into the inner workings of such institutions. The patient groups involved in the running of the alternative institutions described in Chapter 1 also arguably qualify as patient-reformers.

In the late 1960s and 1970s, however, a new and more organised patient movement emerged—one led by patients, often but not exclusively part of a countercultural milieu, and generally hostile to medical authority, including the radical and anti-psychiatrists.[68] The liberatory goals of these groups reflected the revolutionary ethos of the era, as well as the desire to reclaim 'mad' identities from clinical control.[69] Still, the typology of patient activism was and remains diverse. A 'survivor' movement emphasises patients' traumatic suffering at the hands of clinicians.[70] Groups such as the Hearing Voices movement seek to reconceptualise the experience of psychosis.[71] Finally, 'service-user' groups often work within the mental health care system, sometimes in a formalised way, to help improve it, reflecting the disability rights paradigm 'nothing about us, without us.'[72] The advent of 'mad studies' in the academy—a discipline that aims to be both 'survivor-led and theoretically grounded'—has also done much to refocus scholars' attention on the importance of attending to patient voices in the phenomenon they study, generate new methodological insights, as well as forging important links with other forms of critical scholarship (most notably in disability studies).[73] Nevertheless, charges that mad studies have become 'elitist, academicised, racialised,' merely reproducing the concerns of the Global North, in their way continue the radical legacy of the 1960s and 1970s and are an insistent rebuke to clinical and academic certitudes.[74]

Controversies over sexuality and race and the rise of mad activism were emblematic of a larger push during the 1960s and early 1970s to foreground the importance of sociopolitical factors in understanding the production of mental illness. However, as with the advent of post-traumatic stress disorder discussed in Chapter 3, the ultimate results of this advocacy were ambiguous. In attacking entrenched Freudian precepts, critics indirectly bolstered the biomedicalisation of psychiatry and mental health that was gathering pace in the post-war decades. As we have seen in Chapter 2, while biomedical accounts of mental distress need not disregard sociopolitical or cultural factors completely, the overall effect has been to subordinate these considerations to more explicitly neuro-biological mechanisms, so that the case for their relevance to understandings of mental health must be constantly re-prosecuted. The COVID-19 pandemic provides a very recent example of this tendency insofar as it has reanimated discussions about the social determinants of physical and mental health, highlighting in particular the significant racial disparities in health outcomes. In the next chapter, I explore how these contemporary sociopolitical critiques are also connected to 'psychopolitical' critiques of capitalism.

Notes

1 See for example Matt Smith, *The First Resort: The History of Social Psychiatry in the United States* (Columbia University Press, 2023); Michael Straub, *Madness Is Civilization: When the Diagnosis Was Social, 1948–1980* (University of Chicago Press, 2011); and Rhodri Hayward, 'The Invention of the Psychosocial: An Introduction', *History of the Human Sciences* 25, no. 5 (2012): 3–12 and the entire special issue that follows.

2 For an overview see Nancy Tomes, 'Historical Perspectives on Women and Mental Illness,' in *Women, Health, and Medicine in America: a historical handbook*, ed. Rima D. Apple (Garland Publishing, 1990), 143–72.

3 For overviews see Amy Milne-Smith, 'Gender and Madness in Nineteenth-century Britain', *History Compass* 20, no. 11 (2022): e12754; Elaine Showalter, *The Female Malady* (Virago, 1987); Mark Micale, *Hysterical Men: The Hidden History of Male Nervous Illness* (Harvard University Press, 2008); and Andrew Scull, *Hysteria: The Disturbing History* (Oxford University Press, 2012).

4 See for example Clare Shaw and Gillian Proctor, 'Women at the Margins: A Critique of the Diagnosis of Borderline Personality Disorder', *Feminism & Psychology* 15, no. 4 (2005): 483–90 and Jane M. Ussher, 'The Construction and Lived Experience of Women's Distress: Positioning Premenstrual Change as Psychiatric Illness', in *The Madness of Women: Myth and Experience* (Routledge, 2011), 153–84.

5 See Lisa Appignanesi and John Forrester, *Freud's Women* (Virago Press, 1992); they distinguish between the misogynistic 'theorising' Freud and the more 'conventional' and sympathetic 'interpreting' Freud. See also Nathan G. Hale, *The Rise and Crisis of Psychoanalysis in the United States: Freud and the Americans, 1917–1985* (Oxford University Press, 1995), 40–43.

6 See Dorothy Ross, 'Freud and the Vicissitudes of Modernism in the United States, 1940–1980', in *After Freud Left: A Century of Psychoanalysis in America*, ed. John Burnham (Chicago University Press, 2012), 185–88; Mari Jo Buhle, 'Feminists versus Freud', in *Feminism and Its Discontents: A Century of Struggle with Psychoanalysis* (Harvard University Press, 1998), 206–39; and Hale, *Rise and Crisis of Psychoanalysis*, 345–48.

7 Buhle, *Feminism and Its Discontents*, 238; for a helpful overview of Friedan's thought see Rebecca Jo Plant, *Mom: The Transformation of Motherhood in Modern America* (University of Chicago Press, 2010), 146–77.

8 Phyllis Chesler, *Women and Madness* (Avon, 1972). On the modalities of feminist therapy see Straub, *Madness Is Civilization*, 153–59. On the relationship between feminist and radical critiques of psychiatry during this period see Lucas Richert, *Break on Through*, 28–33 and '"Therapy Means Political Change, Not Peanut Butter": American Radical Psychiatry, 1968–1975', *Social History of Medicine* 27, no. 1 (2014): 112–13. For advocacy around the professional position of women within American psychiatry following the APA's establishment of a Task Force on Women see Rebecca Z. Solomon, 'Women in Psychiatry', *AJP* 130, no. 10 (1973): 1136–37 and the special section on 'Women in Psychiatry and Medicine' that follows. For female psychiatrists' advocacy

around revisions to the *Diagnostic and Statistical Manual* see Decker, *The Making of DSM-III*, 217–22.

9 On this see Herzog, *Cold War Freud*, 56–86, particularly 58–62.

10 See for example *A Global History of Sexual Science, 1880–1960*, ed. Veronika Fuechtner, Douglas E. Haynes and Ryan M. Jones (University of California Press, 2018) and *Histories of Sexuality: Between Science and Politics*, ed. Alain Giami and Sharman Levinson (Palgrave Macmillan, 2021).

11 On the ambivalences of the gender dysphoria diagnosis, see Eric Yarbrough, 'The Gender Dysphoria Diagnosis', in *Transgender Mental Health* (American Psychiatric Association Publishing, 2018), 91–110. For historical antecedents of current diagnostic categories see Diederik F. Janssen, '*Melancholia Scytharum*: The Early Modern Psychiatry of Transgender Identification', *History of Psychiatry* 32 (2021): 270–88; Julian Honkasalo, 'When Boys Will *Not* Be Boys: American Eugenics and the Formation of Gender Nonconformity as Psychopathology', *NORMA* 11 (2016): 270–86; and Jules Gill-Peterson, *Histories of the Transgender Child* (University of Minnesota Press, 2018).

12 On the persecution of homosexuals in Cold War America see David K. Johnson, *The Lavender Scare: The Cold War Persecution of Gays and Lesbians in the Federal Government* (University of Chicago Press, 2004) and Margot Canaday, *The Straight State: Sexuality and Citizenship in Twentieth Century America* (Princeton University Press, 2009).

13 On the experience of gay men and women in the US military during the Second World War see Allan Bérubé, *Coming Out Under Fire: The History of Gay Men and Women in World War II*, 2nd ed. (University of North Carolina Press, 2010). Bérubé argues that the persecution of homosexuals in the military became more intense in the post-war period. For a contemporary account see Louis Jolyon West, et al., 'An Approach to the Problem of Homosexuals in the Military Service', *AJP* 115, no. 5 (1958): 392–401. On concerns about sexual psychopathy see Estelle B. Freedman, 'Uncontrollable Desires: The Response to the Sexual Psychopath', *Journal of American History* 74, no. 1 (1987): 83–106.

14 See Naoko Wake, *Private Practices: Harry Stack Sullivan, the Science of Homosexuality, and American Liberalism* (Rutgers University Press, 2011).

15 West, et al., 'An Approach to the Problem of Homosexuals in the Military Service', 400.

16 Karl M. Bowman and Bernice Engle, 'A Psychiatric Evaluation of Laws of Homosexuality', *AJP* 112, no. 8 (1956): 577–83.

17 Ronald Gold, 'Stop It, You're Making Me Sick!', in R.J. Stoller, et al., 'A Symposium: Should Homosexuality Be in the APA Nomenclature?', *AJP* 130, no. 11 (1973): 1212.

18 See account of Manfred S. Guttmacher, 'The Homosexual in Court', *AJP* 112, no. 8 (1956): 591–98.

19 See for example S. Rachman, 'Sexual Disorders and Behaviour Therapy', *AJP* 118, no. 3 (1961): 235–40 and M.P. Feldman and M.J. MacCulloch, 'A Systematic Approach to the Treatment of Homosexuality by Conditioned Aversion: Preliminary Report', *AJP* 121, no. 2 (1964): 167–71. For an encompassing overview see Kate Davison, 'Cold War Pavlov: Homosexual Aversion Therapy in the 1960s', *History of the Human Sciences* 34, no. 1 (2021): 89–119. For the experiences of women subject to this treatment, see Helen Spandler and Sarah Carr, 'Lesbian and Bisexual Women's Experiences of Aversion Therapy in England', *History of the Human Sciences* 35 (2022): 218–36.

20 For the impact of the Kinsey Reports on psychiatric opinion, see Howard Hsueh-Hao Chiang, 'Effecting Science, Affecting Medicine: Homosexuality, the Kinsey Reports, and the Contested Boundaries of Psychopathology in the United States, 1948–1965', *Journal of the History of the Behavioural Science* 44, no. 4 (2008): 300–18.

21 For an overview of these theories see Roel van den Oever, *Mama's Boy: Momism and Homophobia in Postwar American Culture* (Palgrave Macmillan, 2012).

22 Malvina W. Kremer and Alfred H. Rifkin, 'The Early Development of Homosexuality: A Study of Adolescent Lesbians', *AJP* 126, no. 1 (1969): 91–96.

23 On Freud's theorisations of paranoia and homosexuality see Frank J. Sulloway, *Freud: Biologist of the Mind* (Harvard University Press, 1992), 234–35 and 383–84; Franklin S. Klaf and Charles A. Davis, 'Homosexuality and Paranoid Schizophrenia: A Survey of 150 Cases and Controls', *AJP* 116, no. 12 (1960): 1070–75; Robert A. Moore and Melvin L. Selzer, 'Male Homosexuality, Paranoia, and the Schizophrenias', *AJP* 119, no. 8 (1963): 743–47.

24 Evelyn Hooker, 'The Adjustment of the Male Overt Homosexual', *Journal of Projective Techniques* 21, no. 1 (1957): 18; for comparable studies see also Marcel T. Saghir, et al., 'Homosexuality: III. Psychiatric Disorders and Disability in the Male Homosexual', *AJP* 126, no. 8 (1970): 1079–86 and 'Homosexuality. IV. Psychiatric Disorders and Disability in the Female Homosexual', *AJP* 127, no. 2 (1970): 147–54.

25 Irving Bieber, 'Homosexuality—An Adaptive Consequence of Disorder in Psychosexual Development', in Stoller, et al., 'A Symposium: Should Homosexuality Be in the APA Nomenclature?', 1207–16. See also his 'Homosexual Dynamics in Psychiatric Crisis', *AJP* 128, no. 10 (1972): 1268–72.

26 Charles W. Socarides, 'Homosexuality: Findings Derived from 15 Years of Clinical Research' in Stoller, et al., 'A Symposium', 1213; Bieber, 'Homosexuality', 1211.

27 Gold, 'Stop It, You're Making Me Sick!', 1211.

28 Judd Marmor, 'Homosexuality and Cultural Value Systems', in Stoller, et al., 'A Symposium: Should Homosexuality Be in the APA Nomenclature?', 1209; Jack Drescher, 'Judd Marmor, Psychiatry and Homosexuality', *Journal of Gay & Lesbian Psychotherapy* 10, no. 2 (2006): 117–25. Marmor was also supportive of feminist challenges to psychoanalysis's habitual denigration of clitoral sexuality of psychoanalysis: Buhle, *Feminism and Its Discontents*, 225.

29 'Position Statement on Homosexuality and Civil Rights', *AJP* 131, no. 4 (1974): 497.

30 Jack Drescher, 'An Interview with Robert Spitzer', *Journal of Gay and Lesbian Psychotherapy* 7, no. 3 (2003): 97–111. Spitzer uses the term 'nosological diplomacy': 102.

31 For an account of the disturbances in Detroit see Randall B. Woods, *Prisoners of Hope: Lyndon B. Johnson, the Great Society, and the Limits of Liberalism* (Basic Books, 2016), 312–15.

32 P. Lowinger, C. Darrow and F. Huige, 'Case Study of the Detroit Uprising: The Troops and the Leaders', *Arch Gen Psych* 21, no. 1 (1969): 33–38. This was not the only study seeking to measure the effects of the urban disturbances on people's wellbeing. For a later study of the 1967 disturbances in New Haven, see J.R. Greenley, D.P. Gillespie and J.J. Lindenthal, 'A Race Riot's Effect on Psychological Symptoms', *Arch Gen Psych* 32, no. 9 (1975): 1189–95.

33 On Lowinger and the radical psychiatrists see Rickert, *Break on Through*, 45–47.

34 For an earlier statement on the role of clinicians during 'revolutionary social change', see P. Lowinger, 'Sex, Selma and Segregation: A Psychiatrist's View', *International Journal of Social Psychiatry* 14, no. 2 (1968): 119–24.

35 For an account of how these tendencies were reflected in clinical practice see Matthew Gambino, '"These Strangers within Our Gates": Race, Psychiatry and Mental Illness Among Black Americans at St Elizabeths Hospital in Washington, DC, 1900–40', *History of Psychiatry* 19, no. 4 (2008): 387–408. See also Ian Dowbiggin, *Keeping American Sane: Psychiatry and Eugenics in the United States and Canada* (Cornell, 2003) and Michael E. Staub, *The Mismeasure of Minds: Debating Race and Intelligence Between Brown and the Bell Curve* (University of North Carolina Press, 2018).

36 On the contested status of this self-esteem research see G. Bergner, 'Black Children, White Preference: *Brown v. Board*, the Doll Test, and the Politics of Self-Esteem', *American Quarterly* 61, no. 2 (2009): 299–332. On the postwar intersection between psychological thought and racial identity see J. Garcia, *Psychology Comes to Harlem:*

Rethinking the Race Question in Twentieth Century America (Johns Hopkins University Press, 2012).

37 On 'pathologism' see D. Matlin, 'Who Speaks for Harlem? Kenneth B. Clark, Albert Murray, and the Controversies of Black Urban Life', *Journal of American Studies* 46, no. 4 (2012): 875–94. On the at-times fraught influence of white liberal social workers, psychologists and other clinicians see D. Doyle, 'A Load Off Whose Heart? Psychiatry and the Politics of Respectability and Race Representation in Harlem, 1943–45', *Journal of the History of Medicine and Allied Sciences* 75, no. 1 (2019): 54–82. On the role of behavioural psychology in establishing 'locus of control' and 'learned helplessness' as an explanation for social unrest and disadvantage see K. Baistow, 'Problems of Powerlessness: Psychological Explanations of Social Inequality and Civil Unrest in Postwar America', *History of the Human Sciences* 13, no. 3 (2000): 95–116.

38 On the reception of the Moynihan report see J. Hoberman, *Black and Blue: The Origins and Consequences of Medical Racism* (University of California Press, 2012), 141–46 and M.L. Ondaatje, *Black Conservative Intellectuals in Modern America* (University of Pennsylvania Press, 2010), 93–94. For the origins of the 'cultural deprivation' theories long associated with the Moynihan Report see Mical Raz, *What's Wrong with the Poor? Psychiatry, Race, and the War on Poverty* (University of North Carolina Press, 2013).

39 See Raz, *What's Wrong with the Poor?*

40 See A.V. Horowitz and G.N. Grob, 'The Troubled History of Psychiatry's Quest for Specificity', *Journal of Health Politics, Policy & Law* 41, no. 4 (2016): 521–39. For a useful contemporary overview see *Philosophical Issues in Psychiatry: Explanation, Phenomenology, and Nosology*, ed. K.S. Kendler and J. Parnas (Johns Hopkins University Press, 2008). On the controversy over psychiatric evidence at the trial of Kennedy's killer, see 'Psychiatrist Concedes Sirhan Has "Substantial Mental Illness"', *The New York Times*, 4 April 1969, 31.

41 For accounts of community mental health programmes trialled in Black urban communities see J.N. Chappel and R.S. Daniels, 'Home Visiting in a Black Urban Ghetto', *AJP* 126, no. 10 (1970): 1455–60; Jacob R. Fishman and John McCormack, '"Mental Health Without Walls": Community Mental Health in the Ghetto', *AJP* 126, no. 10 (1970): 1461–67.

42 On the health activism of the Black Panther Party see A. Nelson, *Body and Soul: The Black Panther Party and the Fight Against Medical Discrimination* (University of Minnesota Press, 2011). On civil rights activism in the medical community see B. Hoffman, 'Health Care Reform and Social Movements in the United States', *American Journal of Public Health* 93, no. 1 (2003): 75–85; V. Burrows and B. Berney, 'Creating Equal Health Opportunity: How the Medical Civil Rights Movement and the Johnson Administration Desegregated US Hospitals', *Journal of American History* 105, no. 4 (2019): 885–91.

43 For overviews of these controversies, see Decker, *The Making of DSM-III*, 31–33 and 217–22, and Herzog, *Cold War Freud*, 560–86.

44 See 'Position Statement on Alternatives to Violence', *AJP* 126, no. 10 (1970): 1550. For additional contemporary treatments of violence in the psychiatric literature see F.W. Ilfeld, 'Overview of the Causes and Prevention of Violence', *Arch Gen Psych* 20, no. 6 (1969): 675–89; K. Menninger, 'New Violence and the New Psychiatry', *Bulletin of the Menninger Clinic* 32, no. 6 (1968): 341–54; and *Violence and the Struggle for Existence*, ed. D.N. Daniels, et al. (Little, Brown and Company, 1970).

45 I. Philips, et al., 'The Psychiatrist, the APA, and Social Issues: A Symposium', *AJP* 128, no. 6 (1971): 677.

46 'Official Actions: Report of the Trustees' Policy Meeting March 1971', *AJP* 128, no. 3 (1971): 386.

47 'Editor's Notebook: Aggression and Violence', *AJP* 128, no. 4 (1971): 474.

48 By 1965 there were an estimated 300 Black psychiatrists out of a workforce of 17,000, and only four Black psychoanalysts in the entire country: Hoberman, *Black and Blue*, 147. On the impediments to Black physicians receiving speciality training, especially in the South, as well as the question of equitable access to medical training more broadly, see K.K. Thomas, *Deluxe Jim Crow: Civil Rights and American Health Policy, 1935–1954* (University of Georgia Press, 2011), especially 208–28. The desegregation of state psychiatric hospitals was implemented unevenly. In Alabama, for example, desegregation was only mandated after a US District Court ruling in February 1969. See K. Smith, '"A Rather Straightforward Problem": Unravelling Networks of Segregation in Alabama's Psychiatric Hospitals, 1966–1972', in *Viral Networks: Connecting Digital Humanities and Medical History*, ed. E.T. Ewing and K. Randall (Virginia Tech Publishing, 2018), 31–58.

49 See 'Position Statement on the Training of Minority Psychiatrists', *AJP* 128, no. 2 (1971): 257. On the BPA, see T. D'Arrigo, 'On Its 50th Anniversary, BPA Looks Back on History and Ahead to Future', *Psychiatric News* 54, no. 10 (2019): 10.

50 B.E. Jones, et al., 'Problems of Black Psychiatric Residents in White Training Institutes', *AJP* 127, no. 6 (1970): 798–803, 799.

51 For a discussion of anger as a racially mediated form of political capital see D.L. Phoenix, *The Anger Gap: How Race Shapes Emotion in Politics* (Cambridge University Press, 2019).

52 This is not to endorse the now-disputed dichotomy between the civil rights movement and the Black Power movement but, rather, to emphasise the politics of public perception. On revisions to this dichotomy see P.E. Joseph, 'Introduction: Towards a Historiography of the Black Power Movement', in *The Black Power Movement: Rethinking the Civil Rights-Black Power Era*, ed. P.E. Joseph (Routledge, 2006), 1–25.

53 W. Grier and P. Cobbs, *Black Rage* (Basic Books, 1968), 178.

54 K.B. Clark, 'As Old as Human Cruelty', *The New York Times*, 22 September 1968, 373; on Clark's alleged pathologism see Matlin, 'Who Speaks for Harlem?', 878–79.

55 K.B. Clark, *Dark Ghetto: Dilemmas of Social Power* (Harper and Row, 1965), 16.

56 W.E.B. Du Bois, *Black Reconstruction in America: An Essay Toward a History of the Part which Black Folk Played in the Attempt to Reconstruct Democracy in America, 1860–1880* (Russell and Russell, [1935] 1966), 700–01. For a discussion of Du Bois' characterisation of whiteness as a 'proprietary orientation' see E. Myers, 'Beyond the Psychological Wage: Du Bois on White Dominion', *Political Theory* 47, no. 1 (2019): 6–31.

57 See Frantz Fanon, *Wretched of the Earth*, trans. Constance Farrington (Penguin, [1961] 1967), 41: '[T]he settler makes history; his life is an epoch, an Odyssey. He is the absolute beginning . . . The settler makes history and is conscious of making it.'

58 Clark, *Dark Ghetto*, 227–28.

59 Jones, et al., 'Problems of Black Psychiatric Residents', 800.

60 Grier and Cobbs, *Black Rage*, 182, 184–87. For a contemporaneous account of racist violence in the South see S. Hackney, 'Southern Violence', *American Historical Review* 74, no. 3 (1969): 906–25, at 924 where the final explanation turns on 'the sense of grievance that is at the heart of the [white] southern identity.'

61 See Sidney H. Hankerson, et al., 'The Intergenerational Impact of Structural Racism and Cumulative Trauma on Depression', *AJP* 179 (2022): 434–40. On intergenerational trauma in Black families see Shytierra Gaston, 'Historical Racist Violence and Intergenerational Harms: Accounts from Descendants of Lynching Victims', *Annals of the American Academy of Political and Social Science* 694 (2021): 78–91. On the question of reparations see Sandro Galea, et al., 'Reparations as a Public Health Priority—A Strategy for Ending Black-White Health Disparities', *New England Journal of Medicine* (2020); Derek Ross Soled, et al, 'The Case for Health Reparations', *Frontiers in Public Health* 9 (2021): 1–6. For an overview of the recurring debates about race and

intelligence see Davide Serpico, 'The Cyclical Return of the IQ Controversy: Revisiting the Lessons of the Resolution on Genetics, Race and Intelligence', *Journal of the History of Biology* 54 (2021): 199–228.

62 J.R. Allen and L.J. West, 'Flight from Violence: Hippies and the Green Rebellion', *AJP* 125, no. 3 (1968): 364–70. On drug use as means of destroying an 'old acculturated self' see H.R. Brickman, 'The Psychedelic "Hip Scene": Return of the Death Instinct', *AJP* 125, no. 6 (1968): 78–84. Brickman also complained about the 'smug psychologizing' of the profession towards 'a fruitful area for serious study' (ibid., 84). See also J. Buckman, 'Social and Medical Aspects of Illicit Use of LSD', *International Journal of Social Psychiatry* 17, no. 3 (1971): 163–76.

63 On 'severely disturbed' students see R.D. Chessick, 'Review: Morton Levitt and Ben Rubenstein: *The Student Revolt: Totem and Taboo Revisited*', *American Journal of Psychotherapy* 25, no. 3 (1971): 493. See also Straub, *Madness is Civilization*, 167–68.

64 H.S. Hughes, 'Emotional Disturbance and American Social Change, 1944–1969', *AJP* 126, no. 1 (1969), 21–28.

65 See J. Suri, '*AHR* Forum: The Rise and Fall of an International Counterculture, 1960–1975', *AHR* 114, no. 1 (2009), 45–68, particularly 47; J.P. Varon, *Bringing the War Home: The Weather Underground, the Red Army Faction, and Revolutionary Violence in the Sixties and Seventies* (University of California Press, 2004) and B.L. Hillman, *Dressing for the Culture Wars: Style and the Politics of Self-Presentation in the 1960s and 1970s* (University of Nebraska Press, 2015), particularly 31–59.

66 P.R. Miller, 'Social Activists and Social Change: The Chicago Demonstrators', *AJP* 126, no. 12 (1970): 1752–59, 1758. This was not the only time activists were used as research subjects: see W.T. Carpenter Jr, N.R. Tamarkin, and D.E. Raskin, 'Emergency Psychiatric Treatment During a Mass Rally: The March on Washington', *AJP* 127, no. 10 (1971): 1327–32.

67 Steffan Blayney, 'Activist Sources and the Survivor Movement', in *Sources in the History of Psychiatry, from 1800 to the Present*, ed. Chris Millard and Jennifer Wallis (Routledge, 2022), 3. But see also Sarah Chaney, 'No "Sane" Person Would Have Any Idea': Patients' Involvement in Late Nineteenth-century British Asylum Psychiatry', *Medical History* 60, no. 1 (2016): 37–53.

68 On this point see Geoffrey Reaume, 'How is Mad Studies Different from Anti-Psychiatry and Critical Psychiatry?', in *The Routledge International Handbook of Mad Studies*, ed. Peter Beresford and Jasna Russo (Routledge, 2021), 98–107.

69 See for example the account of the West German Socialist Patients' Collective (SPK) in Beatrice Adler-Bolton and Artie Vierkant, *Health Communism* (Verso, 2022), 128–78.

70 For the United States see Nancy Tomes, 'The Patient as a Policy Factor: A Historical Case Study of the Consumer/Survivor Movement in Mental Health', *Health Affairs* (May/June 2006): 720–29.

71 See Angela Woods, 'Voices, Identity, and Meaning-making', *The Lancet* (12 December 2015): 2386–87; Dirk Corstens, et al., 'Emerging Perspectives from the Hearing Voices Movement: Implications for Research and Practice', *Schizophrenia Bulletin* 40 (2014): S285–94; Rory Neirin Higgs, 'Reconceptualizing Psychosis: The Hearing Voices Movement and Social Approaches to Health', *Health and Human Rights Journal* 22, no. 1 (2020): 133–44.

72 For an overview see Diana Rose, 'Service User/Survivor-led Research in Mental Health: Epistemological Possibilities', *Disability & Society* 32 (2017): 773–89.

73 Peter Beresford, 'Introduction', in *The Routledge International Handbook of Mad Studies*, ed. Bereseford and Russo, 1. On methodology and its challenges see Diana Rose and Jayasree Kalathil, 'Power, Privilege and Knowledge: The Untenable Promise of Co-production in Mental "Health"', *Frontiers in Sociology* 4 (2019): 1–11; see also Diana Rose, 'Critical Qualitative Research on "Madness": Knowledge Making and Activism Among Those Designated "Mad"', *Wellcome Open Research* 6 (2021): 1–22. For the

overlap between mad studies and critical disability studies see Tanja Aho, Liat Ben-Moshe and Leon J. Hilton, 'Mad Futures: Affect/Theory/Violence', *American Quarterly* 69, no. 2, (2017): 291–302.

74 Beresford, 'Introduction', 9. For thoughtful treatment of whether Mad Studies belongs inside or outside the academy see Richard A. Ingram, 'A Genealogy of the Concept of "Mad Studies"', in *The Routledge International Handbook of Mad Studies*, ed. Bereseford and Russo, 93–97.

6

MARKETS

The activists of the 1960s and 1970s who argued for the recognition of the impact of the sociopolitical on the production of mental illness did so from an anti-authoritarian standpoint that positioned psychiatry as a powerful instrument of oppression embedded in a wider system of social control. While these critics frequently used psychiatric concepts to paint mainstream society as 'mad,' the ultimate result of these efforts was clinical reform: changes to diagnostic schemas, clinical language and therapeutic practice, initiatives that ultimately strengthened the new biological psychiatry. Nevertheless, these sociopolitical commentaries demonstrated the possibilities of mobilising psychiatric concepts as a means of broader critique. In this final chapter, I outline another iteration of this tendency, albeit one with substantial antecedents: the use of psychiatry and mental health to characterise and critique capitalism itself. While I draw on various Marxist or Marxist-adjacent interpretations, this is not an exclusively Marxist analysis, as will become apparent from the discussion below.[1] Equally, I am not arguing that psychiatric distress is exclusive to capitalist societies. Instead, what I want to suggest is that the psychologised critiques I cover here disclose a common conviction that capitalism is constituted beyond the abstract—that its human effects are the result of human actions, and theorising the psychic toll of these interactions is one way of measuring their consequences. My analysis is in three parts: first, it considers various formulations of a distinctively capitalist 'psychopolitics,' in which the psychic life of subjects, including their mental health, is positioned as irretrievably intertwined with, and thus governed by, the logic of the market; second, it considers one instantiation of this psychopolitics via what I designate as the psychiatrisation of work, and in particular the notion of 'burnout'; and third, it considers the way new digital technologies might incentivise new markets for mental health care.

DOI: 10.4324/9780429351464-7

While 'psychopolitics' can refer to a 'general relationship' between politics and the mental health system, here it denotes the relationship between political economy and the psyche.[2] This chapter thus draws on similar themes to those of the philosopher Byung-Chul Han, whose works *The Burnout Society* (2015) and *Psychopolitics* (2017) are heavily psychologised accounts of constrained subjectivity under neoliberalist late capitalism. In the former, Han argues that rather than 'disciplinary subjects,' we are now 'achievement-subjects,' creatures of endless striving, not so much as selves as 'projects,' caught in a forever recursion in which 'the achievement-subject exploits itself until it burns out.'[3] In the latter, Han proposes that such 'allo-exploitation' renders neoliberalism self-sustaining, and that this dynamic is strongly abetted by pervasive digital technologies that 'intervene in psychic processes in a prospective fashion,' not merely surveilling the individual but pre-emptively 'steering' them towards the reproduction of neoliberalist logic.[4] While Han argues that these formulations are necessary updates to Foucauldian notions of biopolitical, disciplinary societies, the scholarship I survey here suggests that this rupture can be overstated and that Han's formulations not only underplay Foucault's insights into the neoliberalist demands on the subject (*homo oeconomicus*, who is now 'an entrepreneur of himself'), but that both sit within a broader literature that theorises capitalism as producing a totalising relationship between the psyche and the market.[5] Over time, however, this relationship has shifted from the overt depredations of industrial capitalism towards the complicity required by neoliberalism: from labouring *under* capitalism to an equally oppressive labouring *with* capitalism.

While an obvious starting point is the attempted conciliations of Marx and Freud that characterised the interwar period, there are some important precursors worth rehearsing. First, there are the actual material effects of capitalism on the management of madness and the development of psychiatry and related disciplines. As discussed in Chapter 1, the transformations wrought by industrial capitalism in nineteenth-century Britain, and in particular growing official interest in the proliferating metropolitan underclass, had a profound effect on the development of asylums and the professionalisation of psychiatry. Urbanisation, mechanisation, and their related social effects—weakened communal bonds, increased poverty, time discipline and its demands, increasing rates of alcoholism and neurosyphilis (often precursors to institutionalisation)—simultaneously decreased the capacity of families to care for insane family members while also swelling the ranks of the insane in urban settings. This also produced new typologies of nervous disorder, such as 'railway spine' and neurasthenia, as well as sociological accounts of the city that anticipated similarly psychological interpretations of industrial capitalism.[6] These accounts emphasised speed and atomisation: Émile Durkheim's notion of 'anomie' was predicated on the breakdown of rules, disciplines and structures brought about by industrialisation and urbanisation; Georg Simmel's new 'metropolitan type of individuality' on 'the *intensification of nervous stimulation* which results from the swift and uninterrupted change of outer and inner stimuli.'[7]

Cognate discussions of capitalism's 'rationality' also anticipate and reflect a psychologised interpretation of capitalist economics. Wendy Brown's influential interpretation of contemporary neoliberalism, for example, argues that neoliberalism promulgates an 'order of normative reason,' one that overturns the liberal 'rationality' of exchange elaborated by Adam Smith and Jeremy Bentham, by substituting a new 'governing rationality extending a specific formulation of economic values, practices, and metrics to every dimension of human life.'[8] Marx also regarded capitalists as practising a kind of rationality in their attitude towards the circular and 'unceasing movement of profit-making,' which made the capitalist a 'rational miser' and the miser 'merely a capitalist gone mad.'[9] And, while sceptical of Marx's economism, Max Weber offered similar arguments in *The Protestant Ethic and the Spirit of Capitalism* (1904–5)—a psychologised genealogy of capitalism written in the wake of Weber's own nervous breakdown. Here, he proposed that the Calvinist doctrine of predestination yoked sublimated spiritual terror to an 'ascetic compulsion to save,' producing an ethos of self-consciously rational capitalism, in which '[u]nlimited greed for gain' was understood as an 'irrational impulse.'[10] The spending of profit for personal enjoyment was illegitimate; saving profit in order to create more profit was not. This exacting, steady but also self-denying accumulation of profit was central to early modern mercantile capitalism and, argued Weber, persisted as a sublimated psychic residue in capitalism's industrial phase, which was also sustained by standardised routines and procedures that governed labour and investment. Personal rationality thus became a more generalised instrumental rationality.[11]

Beginning in the 1920s, theorising the production of this capitalist rationality and its pervasive effects was a central concern of Western Marxism, as adherents sought to understand the aftermath of the revolution in Russia as well as the failed revolutions in Central Europe and elsewhere. Here, what we might call 'totalisation' emerged as a key theme, the effects of which were increasingly psychologised. Georg Lukács' concept of 'reification' proposed that Marx's notion of the 'fetishism of commodities' could be applied not just to social relations but to the 'whole consciousness of man,' resulting in both the fragmentation of experience and the elevation of a '"phantom objectivity", an autonomy that seems so strictly rational and all-embracing as to conceal every trace of its fundamental nature: the relation between people.'[12] Theorists of the Frankfurt School more deliberately looked beyond prevailing understandings of orthodox Marxism and toward psychoanalysis—a worldview that also traded in universals, as we have seen in previous chapters—to expand the bounds of the political, producing critical accounts of art, music, literature, and mass culture as emblematic of social relations under capitalism. With the rise of Nazism sending many key theorists into exile in the United States, these attempted conciliations of Freud and Marx also offered a means of comprehending the rise of fascism in interwar Europe and the cataclysm of the Second World War.[13] While works like Erich Fromm's *Escape from Freedom* (1941) and Theodor Adorno's *The Authoritarian Personality* (1950) offered explicitly psychologised accounts of fascism's malign appeal, other accounts advanced more encompassing theories that emphasised capitalism's hegemonic and thus totalising qualities, renderings that anticipate the kind of 'allo-exploitation' Han invokes. In the *Dialectic of Enlightenment* (1947), for example, Max Horkheimer and Adorno pointed to the triumph of pervasive 'instrumental reason' as constraining the possibilities of human freedom and rationalising domination and exploitation, so that subjects collude in their own oppression. Herbert Marcuse's *One-Dimensional Man* (1964) also anticipated the contemporary characterisation of neoliberalism's totalising psychic effects by proposing that the central political conundrum of Leftist politics was how to undo what was, in the end, the subject's conquest of itself.[14]

Echoes of this totalisation theme can also be heard in and around postmodern theory. In *Anti-Oedipus* (1972) and *A Thousand Plateaus* (1980), the philosopher Gilles Deleuze and the psychiatrist Félix Guattari proposed 'schizoanalysis'—a 'task' that 'goes by way of destruction'—as the prime means to counter 'the capitalist machine and the pathological character of its rationality,' as well as to excavate a 'de-opedialised,' 'deterritorialised,' polyphonic consciousness free from psychoanalytic strictures.[15] Deleuze and Guattari proposed that humans were best understood as 'desiring machines,' whose liberation could be found in a radical anti-identitarianism that amplified interconnections, contingencies, and flux—precepts that Guattari had sought to practise at the therapeutic community of La Borde, where he had lived and worked since the 1950s.[16] Yet while Deleuze and Guattari used psychologised language, the relationship between their analysis and actual clinical practice is not clear—in particular, how the reader ought to understand Deleuze and Guattari's mobilisation of schizophrenia, the related 'schizoanalysis' and the relationship of these concepts to capitalism. Critics have repeatedly charged that, like some of the anti-psychiatrists, Deleuze and Guattari merely romanticised schizophrenia for rhetorical purposes.[17] A counter-interpretation is that their intention is strictly metaphorical, underscoring the cleaving of the 'psy' language of the academy from its clinical origins—a phenomenon also seen in Frederic Jameson's invocation, following Lacan, of postmodernity's 'schizophrenic' temporalities, and Jean Baudrillard's notion of a 'new' schizophrenia comprised of interminable, networked 'over-proximity.'[18] Regardless, the emergent form of capitalism Deleuze and Guattari invoked—globalised, borderless, forever-circulating, forever 'territorialising' individuals, who can only resist via constant effortful acts of schizoanalytic destruction—suggests totalisation of similar intensity to the formulations of the Frankfurt School and their predecessors, as well as the usefulness of capitalist psychopolitics as means of illumination and critique.

The psychiatrisation of work

For its proponents, the generalised psychopolitics outlined above produces specific expressions in the world of work. As with the relationship between capitalism and the history of the asylum, work is relevant to the history of psychiatry in two broad senses. First, patient labour served important purposes within asylums, where it was understood as both discipline and therapy. As discussed in Chapter 1, routinised daily work was an important pillar of the moral treatment practised by Samuel Tuke and others. The capacity to work was also a barometer of patients' recovery. More pragmatically, unpaid patient labour was also vital for the actual running of many underfunded—or parsimonious—institutions.[19] More tellingly, over the course of the twentieth century, unemployment was increasingly medicalised, so that chronic unemployment or eccentric work histories might also be cast as a psychopathology—an assumption with parallels in contemporary, psychologised 'workfare' regimes, as critics point out.[20]

Against this tendency to regard work as a therapeutic good is the history of workplaces as quasi-clinical spaces, in which workers but also organisations themselves were understood and managed in psychological terms. A leading example from the early twentieth century is the field of industrial psychology, which rose to prominence in the interwar period and reflected a new popular interest in psychodynamic theories as well as an older tradition of factory medicine. While initially concerned with solving issues like absenteeism and industrial accidents, after the Second World War, this speciality began to address wider concerns like organisational performance by drawing on theories of interpersonal and group behaviour elaborated in wartime contexts.[21] A good example of these developments is the Tavistock Institute of Human Relations, established in 1946 as an offshoot of the psychoanalytically inclined Tavistock Clinic in London, whose clinicians had been closely involved in British wartime psychiatry. As the editors declared in the inaugural issue of the Institute's journal *Human Relations*:

> The recent war gave urgency and opportunity for work on large scale problems, and also gave experience in handling the complicated interpersonal and inter-group tensions which new undertakings by specialists within an institution invariably involve.[22]

The political character of this emerging organisational psychology was decidedly ambivalent. During the war, several of the Tavistock clinicians had pursued projects with a broadly social democratic ethos that emphasised devolved authority and group cohesion, such as the rehabilitation of prisoners of war.[23] Yet many of the projects reported in *Human Relations* reinforced existing hierarchies, usually undertaken at the behest of management. One study of female workers at a textile factory in Virginia concluded that management—rattled by worker 'resistance' to new work processes that lowered their piece rates—could overcome this by using 'group meetings in which management effectively communicates the need for change and stimulates group participation in planning the changes.'[24] Other articles investigated techniques for determining workplace morale,[25] workplace accidents as 'motivated forms of withdrawal,'[26] methods of control within organisations[27], and social psychologists as 'agents of social change' in businesses.[28]

While understanding the collective psychology of workers and organisations was the focus of post-war industrial and organisational psychology, in the following decades the shift from industrial to global consumer capitalism, the corresponding increase in people working in 'service' roles, and the decline of unions turned the field away from groups and towards the individual employee as the object of psychologised care and surveillance.[29] The emergence of 'human resource management' (HRM) as both a discrete business function and a field of expert knowledge reflects these developments.[30] Indeed, in many contemporary workplaces HRM specialists now manage both the administration of employees and various 'well-being' initiatives purporting to safeguard employees' mental health (the latter creating a substantial market for external providers).[31] In addition, many large workplaces also offer access to free or subsidised psychological counselling—employee benefits that recognise the prevalence of mental illness in the general population but that also provide moral cover for the kind of distress the workplace may generate.[32]

Yet mental health can also be grounds for criticism and resistance in the workplace. In 2022, the International Labour Organisation Declaration on Fundamental Principles and Rights at Work added a fifth principle—'a safe and healthy working environment'—which can be interpreted as requiring employers to protect workers' psychological health.[33] Renewed interest in the notion of 'burnout'—used by Han, as we have seen, to indicate neoliberalism's destructive effects but also elaborated in various mainstream titles currently on the market—speaks to a similar tendency.[34] As Hannah Proctor has recently argued, burnout can also powerfully evoke the emotional toll of political struggle and defeat.[35] Indeed, the term itself has a telling history, with conceptual links to stress research but also practical origins in the clinical counterculture of the 1960s and 1970s.[36] In a 1974 paper generally credited with popularising the concept, the psychologist Herbert J. Freudenberger argued that burnout was an occupational risk for those working in alternative institutions—the 'free clinics, therapeutic communities, hot lines, crisis intervention centres, women's clinics, gay centres, runaway houses,' all endeavours requiring substantial animating idealism and then sustained personal commitment despite endemic underfunding.[37]

According to Freudenberger, burnout often began with physical symptoms: 'a feeling of exhaustion and fatigue, being unable to shake a lingering cold, suffering from frequent headaches and gastrointestinal disturbances, sleeplessness and shortness of breath.' Then came altered behaviour: angry outbursts, paranoia, risk-taking, depression, isolation. Those suffering from burnout had usually been working 'too much, too long and too intensely,' but there were psychological dynamics as well: high ideals followed by dashed hopes, as well as boredom once the crises of the heady early days were over:

> If your idealism, the very motivation that led you to come into an institution as a volunteer, has been lost, then the burn-out has also within it the dynamics of mourning. Something has died. There has been a real loss.[38]

Freudenberger also argued that work in therapeutic communities and other alternative institutions was unusually exacting, requiring an extraordinary level of emotional commitment and openness. Workers in such establishments 'must be ready to give haircuts [verbal reprimands], probes, to call encounters, to have encounters called on them, to rap, to receive criticism, to be sympathetic, to be firm, to have patience, to ignore their own discomforts and preferences almost without respite.'[39] While there were practical interventions that might ameliorate some of the effects, such as careful attention to rosters, Freudenberger warned that the nature of the work made it impossible to avoid burnout completely.

As with the depoliticisation of PTSD discussed in Chapter 3 and the sociopolitical critiques outlined in Chapter 5, burnout was soon separated from its roots in the counterculture. Research by the social psychologist Christina Maslach applied 'burnout' to human services more broadly, and then to white-collar workplaces in general, measurable by a diagnostic tool—the Maslach Burnout Inventory (MBI). By the 1980s, Maslach and also Freudenberger had written books on burnout for the popular market, and, regardless of their intentions, the concept began to take on a distinctly individualised, 'self-help' orientation.[40] Now, anyone in white-collar employment could burn out, including the dyspeptic executives overseeing it all. The political implications shifted: this was not about the stress of working with vulnerable people for little pay, but about employees' own vulnerabilities and their capacity to properly manage workplace stress.

Renewed academic interest in burnout, particularly in those professions most affected by the COVID-19 pandemic, may go some way to repoliticising the concept, though whether this will result in lasting change is difficult to say.[41] Almost by definition burnout decimates the energy required for collective action. Recent studies into 'physician burnout' emphasise this: how difficult it is for already-exhausted doctors to 'initiate, sustain, and complete interventions to improve their well-being,' perhaps more so in a profession where unionisation is controversial.[42] The term's imprecision does not help.[43] While it is absent from the *Diagnostic and Statistical Manual* (DSM), in 2019 a new expanded definition of burnout was added to the WHO's ICD-11, which listed it as an 'occupational phenomenon' rather than a medical condition, the result of 'chronic workplace stress that has not been successfully managed'—although, crucially, it is not clear by whom.[44]

Alongside burnout the urgent concerns of the present may yet prompt the formulation of new types of psychopathies. One example is the use of psychiatric concepts to describe the psychological effects of environmental damage and a looming climate catastrophe (and, conversely, to pathologise climate activists as mentally ill).[45] 'Solastalgia,' a term coined by the Australian philosopher Glenn Albrecht, describes 'the homesickness we feel while still at home' and is brought about by irrevocable changes to the sufferer's home environment. For Albrecht, this distress was evident in communities impacted by the large open-cut coal mines that now dominate the Upper Hunter region of New South Wales, not far from where this book was written, as well as in the experience of Indigenous people in the aftermath of dispossession.[46] Albrecht has gone on to coin other psychologically inflected neologisms, arguing that humanity needs a new vocabulary to rethink its relationship to the natural world and the distress that results from its destruction.[47] Moves to conceptualise 'planetary health' display a similar impulse.[48]

Digital markets and mental health

Han's articulation of a 'digital psychopolitics' can be linked to other questions about the intersections of mental health, the market and the digital sphere, which encompass both the possibility of harm and new therapeutic possibilities. The potential harms are not just overt instances—cyberbullying, for example, or the facilitation of porn and gambling addictions—but the cumulative effects of constant connectivity or sustained immersion in social media. Particular attention has been paid to rising rates of mental illness amongst adolescents, especially young women, seemingly correlated to the advent of social media and the iPhone. Yet establishing causation is complex, not least because these technologies are embedded within complex and individuated social worlds. For example, it is difficult to separate social media content from the conditions under which it is consumed; some forms of social media might be helpful for some adolescents some of the time; adolescents with poor mental health might be more likely to use social media than their peers (and with the possibility of also being *helped* by online support groups).[49] The apparent susceptibility of girls to these mental health problems is also hard to disentangle from its broader social context, as well as a history of suspicion about female fragility.

Simultaneously, new forms of digital therapeutics also invite scrutiny and speculation. The COVID-19 pandemic accelerated developments in digital health that had been brewing since the early 2000s, when it was recognised that these technologies could improve the capacity of certain patients—those living remotely, or with mobility issues, or with conditions that render them housebound, such as agoraphobia—to access mental health treatment.[50] Prior to the pandemic, many of the digital developments in mental health treatments focused on Cognitive Behavioural Therapy (CBT)—as we saw in a previous chapter, a modality particularly suited to 'manualisation.'[51] The potential for CBT conducted online to improve accessibility and reduce costs became apparent as internet use became more widespread. A 2008 editorial in the *British Journal of Psychiatry* emphasised the financial benefits of administering online CBT cheaply and at scale, arguing that given the reported rates of mild to moderate depression, '[e]ven a minor improvement of depression symptoms could have a large impact on the disease burden of depression if the treatment is safe and cheap.'[52] Post-pandemic this imperative remains: the World Health Organization, for example, cites digital technologies as a means to extend mental health care for people in low- and middle-income countries, where smartphone ownership is increasing.[53] In the Global North, too, governments are also interested in expanding digital interventions to address service gaps without the need for costly spending on physical infrastructure, such as in rural areas.[54]

Yet, predictably, the private sector has a keen interest in these technologies as well. While generic 'wellness' was already heavily monetised in online spaces, the pandemic disruptions and lockdowns supercharged demand for mental health services that could now only be delivered remotely. In 2021 investors channelled a reported $4.8 billion into digital mental health start-ups, many of them app-based ventures like BetterHelp, which focuses on online therapy, and Cerebral, which prescribes pharmaceuticals.[55]

Now even newer technologies offer further possibilities for digital therapeutics and their monetisation. In particular, the public release of the ChatGPT platform in November 2022 has prompted renewed attention to the potential applications of Artificial Intelligence (AI) in psychiatry and related disciplines, an interest that has been building for the last decade and is closely tied to developments in computational psychiatry.[56] Whereas mental health apps seek to streamline patient–clinician interactions, advances in natural language processing (NLP), machine learning (ML), and generative AI suggest three possibilities for the future of psychiatry I will discuss here: new forms of explanation, new powers of prediction, and new capacities for automation.

Speaking generally, explanatory modelling theorises mental illness as 'malfunctions' of the brain's computational processes and contends that both normal and abnormal functioning can be modelled by applying statistical reasoning to hypothesised systems of brain functioning. The resulting models then provide mechanistic explanations for the production of psychiatric disorders. Without rehearsing the history of the 'brain-as-computer' hypothesis and its various controversies here, advocates for these techniques regard them as offering a way through the conceptual impasses of descriptive diagnoses, something evident in the 'enormous explanatory gap' generated by 'a lack of appropriate intermediate levels of description that bind ideas articulated at the molecular level to those expressed at the level of descriptive clinical entities, such as schizophrenia, depression and anxiety.'[57] Somewhat ironically, this gap has been exacerbated by the success of psychotropic drugs in relieving symptoms because, as we saw in Chapter 2, their therapeutic effects do not explain the mechanisms that produce the symptoms they ameliorate. By contrast, proponents of computational modelling regard it as a means of concretising the cognitive 'bridge' between 'the molecular and the phenomenological,' on the basis that decision-making (normal and abnormal) is the proving ground of mental illness. Thus, 'if the psychology and neurobiology of normative decision-making can be characterised and parameterised via a multi-level computational framework, it will be possible to understand the many ways in which decision-making can go wrong.'[58]

In contrast to explanatory models, predictive applications use machine learning techniques to process vast clinical datasets in order to refine diagnostic categories, theorise the relationships between symptoms, and predict treatment responses and other patient behaviours. Here, potential clinical applications are immediately apparent. The existence of vast digitised datasets generated by activity on social media, electronic health records, or the metrics produced by wearable technology allows ML systems to run prediction algorithms with uses for individual patients and across vulnerable cohorts. Patients with bipolar disorder, for example, may be able to use such tools in consultation with their doctor to predict and manage the onset of a manic or depressive episode.[59] Doctors may be able to better predict which patients would most benefit from certain medications.[60] Similarly, such predictive systems may be able to both simulate and analyse the disordered language some theorists argue is characteristic of schizophrenia's 'formal thought disorder' and thus predict the onset of psychosis.[61] There is also much hope that these techniques will be useful for suicide prevention—a long-time problem for clinicians, given the incentive for suicidal patients to conceal their intentions, and a conceptual problem, in the sense that is difficult to write algorithms that predict statistically rare if devastating events.[62] Potential applications include better data gathering on attempted and completed suicides, the flagging of important broader sociodemographic factors (such as community of residence), and the ability to practice more directed outreach.[63]

New suicide prevention measures have important implications for governments given the politically sensitive issue of high suicide rates in the veteran community—numbers that appear resistant to the many programs, resources and other interventions aimed at destigmatising mental illness in the military.[64] The United States Department of Veterans Affairs now uses such a prediction algorithm to more closely monitor veterans deemed at the highest risk of suicide.[65] But there are some unanswered questions here, including concerns about privacy, surveillance, and autonomy, that are part of a broader set of 'gaps' that are common to digital mental health tools.[66] How will clinicians use such information in relation to their own expertise and judgement? Which cohorts will benefit from such tools, beyond the politically visible veteran community? And, importantly, how will patients identified by such algorithms respond? This is particularly relevant in relation to suicide prevention, where interventions can have complex and even perverse outcomes. Few high-risk patients in a survey group providing feedback on the Veterans Affairs trial of outreach scripts reported adverse responses, such as an increased feeling of hopelessness.[67] Yet whether this will be replicated in larger cohorts is unclear. More broadly, AI tools also add potential algorithmic bias to already biased health systems.[68] For example, the algorithmically derived diagnoses of 'formal thought disorder' discussed above may incorrectly categorise bilingual speakers as pre-psychotic if the training data are drawn only from native speakers.[69] Perennial controversies over diagnoses may also mean that, in the words of a recent review, 'labels of disease states may not be specific enough to yield AI algorithms with high sensitivity and specificity.'[70] 'Explainable' AI will therefore be imperative to protect the rights of patients and retain human clinical control.

The final implication for AI in mental health relates to automation, and in particular automated therapy, which has loomed as a possibility since the mid-1960s, when the MIT computer scientist Joseph Weizenbaum released the now-famous

ELIZA program. ELIZA 'decomposed' the text typed by a user and then 'reassembled' it as a question or statement according to a set of predetermined rules.[71] This resulted in human–machine 'conversations' that approximated what Weizenbaum described as 'Rogerian' psychotherapy—a 'non-directive' approach developed by the American psychologist Carl Rogers, in which the therapist supports but does not direct or instruct the patient.[72] For Weizenbaum, such encounters were 'one of the few examples of categorised dyadic natural language communication in which one of the participating pair is free to assume the pose of knowing almost nothing of the real world.' This 'not-knowingness' was central to ELIZA's conversational style, which quickly became repetitive and circular—characteristics that, to Weizenbaum, made ELIZA's limits abundantly clear. He was therefore unnerved by the tendency of human users to attribute outsize weight and meaning to their interactions with the program, as though they were participating in real conversations. In addition, he was concerned by what he interpreted as the hubris of the computer science community regarding the possibilities of machine intelligence. He spent much of the rest of his career warning about the dangers of AI and other forms of technological overreach.[73]

Yet other researchers felt precisely the opposite. In the weeks before Weizenbaum's first ELIZA paper appeared, the Stanford psychiatrist Kenneth Mark Colby (who we first met in Chapter 4 criticising the racialised psychiatry of J.C. Carothers) and his colleagues published an account of a similar program in the *Journal of Nervous and Mental Disease*. The Stanford team had also 'written a computer program which can conduct psychotherapeutic dialogue,' a system that was 'conceptually equivalent' to ELIZA, but with the express purpose of eliciting 'a communicative experience *intended* to be psychotherapeutic' (my italics).[74] Although '[a]lmost everyone who has participated in these dialogues reports that he comes to feel annoyed and frustrated by the program's responses,' the Stanford team believed that with further refinement the program might be useful for 'mental hospitals and psychiatric centres suffering a shortage of therapists.'[75] Indeed, the new time-sharing capacity of modern computers would allow 'several hundred patients an hour' to undergo this kind of automated therapy, freeing up the human therapist to be 'a much more efficient man.' For Colby, far from demonstrating the limits of such systems, human interactions with programs like ELIZA invoked a new therapeutic future, in which the uncertainties of psychoanalysis, with which Colby had become disillusioned, or the biases of a clinician like Carothers, would no longer intrude.[76]

Weizenbaum was predictably critical of the notion of machine therapists, arguing that they could only offer 'impoverished' forms of simulated care.[77] Yet the kind of machine–human interactions Colby proposed in his 1966 paper were not so far removed from other attempts to automate therapeutic encounters. As we have seen, cognitive therapy and rational therapy could be streamlined by way of worksheets—analogue forerunners of contemporary online versions. The increasing availability of audiotape and videotape recorders extended such possibilities further into other cost-effective interventions. In the 1970s, for example, one group of researchers used a combination of film clips and an instructional audiotape to desensitise flight-phobic passengers. These materials were administered not by clinicians but by 'housewives and college students.' According to the authors, this work was significant insofar as it 'combined desensitisation, modelling, and positive reinforcement in a totally automated audiovisual program and was administered by non-professionals who had no contact with the authors.'[78] Similar programs are used in the present: contemporary treatment for agoraphobic patients, for example, continues to use such automated, simulated protocols as a means of exposure therapy.[79]

Colby, for his part, eventually acknowledged some of Weizenbaum's qualms, albeit somewhat elliptically. In a paper published in 1986, he implied that critics of 'computer-assisted psychotherapy' were attacking a strawman, invoking a 'dehumanised' situation in which 'one might see a patient sitting alone in a room and interacting with a computer by means of a keyboard.' This was not the intention, Colby insisted: rather, computer-assisted psychotherapy would be a group exercise—something not apparent in the 1966 paper. In this collective format, groups of patients would sit in a room at their own computer terminal and interact with a 'therapeutic learning program,' interspersed with discussions between the patient and 'a human therapist trained in carrying out the procedures of this method.' The therapist would provide 'human elements of warmth, empathy, humour, and intuition considered desirable in the helping relationship of psychotherapy,' and the presence of the other patients would 'add further human qualities of group support and examples of similar personal problems.'[80]

Several decades on from this clarification, Colby's version of automated therapy appears quaint in the context of our increasingly digitised lives. Given that many people spend much of their time 'sitting alone in a room and interacting with a computer by means of a keyboard,' it is not unreasonable to imagine that generative AI platforms such as ChatGPT may soon become quite normalised as machine therapists, whether as text-based interfaces, disembodied voices, avatars, or embodied 'social' robots.[81] If our reflexive response is like Weizenbaum's, we will dismiss these machine therapists as poor imitations, the predictable outcome of psychiatry conducted for quick profit and at scale. Yet it is worth pausing to consider just what constitutes good therapy. As we saw in Chapter 2, the history of psychiatric treatment offers no easy answers. Despite Weinzenbaum's denunciations, for some patients it may be precisely a chatbot's non-humanness—the fact that it neither judges nor cares—that imparts therapeutic effects.[82] Indeed, some researchers suggest that chatbots could be valuable early screening tools for groups hesitant to disclose mental health concerns to human clinicians, such as serving military personnel.[83] Of course, there are ethical implications to therapy completely stripped of human judgement, as we saw in the concerns about the treatment of morally compromised veterans in the aftermath of the Vietnam War. What this indicates more broadly, however, is the ambivalence that underwrites what the sociologist Sherry Turkle called the 'ELIZA effect'—our propensity to humanise technologies like Weizenbaum's ELIZA program. As we interact with these systems, we become more adept at recognising their limitations, comfort which produces first legitimation, and then normalisation. In the case of ELIZA, this reflected users' perception that psychotherapy had become more cognitive and 'scientific.'[84] New AI-enabled technologies will be subject to the same process.

Conclusion

In this chapter and throughout this book, we have seen examples of the way the market shapes therapeutic spaces and can herald both austerity and largesse. In the private madhouses of eighteenth-century Britain, in the popularity of private psychotherapy in the post-war United States, in the justifications for deinstitutionalisation in Britain, in pharmaceutical companies' ceaseless search for new markets, in venture capital's interest in the possibilities of online therapy, the market delineates and clarifies therapeutic possibilities. Thus, while it is likely that this newer, faster, more automated digital world might democratise some elements of the mental health landscape, it will also radically stratify others. To take a very recent example: in May 2023, researchers at the University of Texas reported that they had developed a non-invasive 'brain–computer interface' capable of acting as a personalised 'language decoder,' able to infer 'the meaning of perceived speech, imagined speech and even silent videos' from an individual's fMRI imaging.[85] This system used a predictive model trained on hours of an individual's fMRI data, collected while the research subject listened to podcasts and watched animated films. Press coverage of the study characterised these procedures as a form of mind-reading—a designation that may, for once, prove accurate.[86] Provided such systems have access to sufficient training data, it may indeed be possible to reconstruct something approximating an individual's silent thoughts.

These are extraordinary findings, with significant implications for patients suffering speech deficits due to brain injuries and other conditions, whose best options are surgically implanted devices (although these are also increasingly utilising AI capabilities).[87] Yet it is also not difficult to think of the potential mental health applications of such a brain–computer interface; for example, the way it might override a total reliance on a clinician's interpretation of the patient's self-report, especially when combined with the explanatory and predictive functions of computational psychiatry described above.[88] Yet in typifying the possibilities of intensely personalised medicine, such technology also raises disquieting questions about accessibility and monetisation, as well as what researchers describe as 'mental privacy.'[89] In the University of Texas study, the research subjects were able to 'resist' the interface by silently performing tasks in an idiosyncratic or unpredictable manner, suggesting that cooperation is necessary to produce a truly accurate decoder for any individual. But given creations often run ahead of their creators, one could easily imagine a more sinister scenario in which such nuance is discarded, and brain–computer interfaces become a new kind of polygraph test, calibrated to a spurious baseline, with deviations from this supposed norm pathologised—or monetised. Even the more trivial applications may end up fuelling new kinds of therapies or reanimating old ones. Perhaps the billionaires who today fly to space will tomorrow sleep in brain scanners and so resurrect the dream interpretation of the psychoanalysts.[90] In offering up the brain to the market, such dreams and nightmares coexist.

Notes

1 For a recent Marxist analysis see Bruce M.Z. Cohen, *Psychiatric Hegemony: A Marxist Theory of Mental Illness* (Palgrave, 2016).
2 For this early generalised use see Milton Greenblatt, 'Towards a Definition of Psychopolitics', *Psychiatric Annals* 5, no. 10 (1975): 393–98; Peter Sedgwick, *Psycho Politics* (Verso, 2022; first published in 1982).
3 Byung-Chul Han, *The Burnout Society*, trans. Erik Butler (Stanford, 2015), 36, 38, 47.
4 Byung-Chul Han, *Psychopolitics: Neoliberalism and New Technologies of Power*, trans. Erik Butler (Verso, 2017), 11, 63.
5 See Han, *Psychopolitics*, 23–28; see Michel Foucault, *The Birth of Biopolitics: Lectures at the Collège de France, 1978–1979*, trans. Graham Burchell (Palgrave, 2008), 226; Caroline Alphin and François Debrix, 'Biopolitics in the "Psychic Realm": Han, Foucault and Neoliberal Psychopolitics', *Philosophy & Social Criticism* 49, no. 4 (2021): 477–91. See also Jason Read, 'A Genealogy of Homo-Economicus: Neoliberalism and the Production of Subjectivity', *Foucault Studies* 6 (2009): 25–36.
6 John Erichsen, *On Railway and Other Injuries of the Nervous System* (Henry C. Lea, 1867); George Beard, 'Neurasthenia, or Nervous Exhaustion', *Boston Medical and Surgical Journal*, 29 April 1869: 217–21.
7 Émile Durkheim, *Suicide: A Study in Sociology*, trans. John A. Spaulding and George Simpson (Free Press, 1951); Georg Simmel, 'The Metropolis and Mental Life', in *The Sociology of Georg Simmel*, ed. Kurt H. Wolff (Free Press, 1950), 409–10.
8 See Wendy Brown, *Undoing the Demos: Neoliberalism's Stealth Revolution* (Zone Books, 2015), 30, 32–34.
9 Karl Marx, *Capital: A Critique of Political Economy, Volume One*, trans. Ben Fowkes (Penguin, 1976), 247–55, particularly 254–55.
10 Weber likely had bipolar disorder: see Fritz Ringer, *Max Weber: An Intellectual Biography* (University of Chicago Press, 2004), 2. On the relationship between Weber's personal context and the writing and publication of *The Protestant Ethic* see ibid., 113–42.
11 Max Weber, *The Protestant Ethic and the Spirit of Capitalism*, trans. Talcott Parsons (Routledge, 2001), xxxi-xxxii, 116; for helpful commentary see Peter Ghosh, *Max Weber and the Protestant Ethic: Twin Histories* (Oxford University Press, 2014).
12 Georg Lukács, 'Reification and the Consciousness of the Proletariat', in *History and Class Consciousness: Studies in Marxist Dialectics*, trans. Rodney Livingstone (Merlin Press, 1971), 83.
13 For general histories of the Frankfurt School see Martin Jay, *The Dialectical Imagination: A History of the Frankfurt School and the Institute for Social Research, 1923–1950* (University of California Press, 1973) and Thomas Wheatland, *The Frankfurt School in Exile* (University of Minnesota Press, 2009).
14 Erich Fromm, *Escape from Freedom* (Avon Books, 1965); Theodor W. Adorno, *The Authoritarian Personality* (Harper & Row, 1950); Max Horkheimer and Theodor W. Adorno, *Dialectic of Enlightenment* (Allen Lane, 1973); Herbert Marcuse,

One-dimensional Man: Studies in the Ideology of Advanced Industrial Society (Routledge, 2002).

15 Gilles Deleuze and Félix Guattari, *Anti-Oedipus: Capitalism and Schizophrenia*, trans. Robert Hurley, Mark Seem and Helen R. Lane (Penguin, 2009), 311; *A Thousand Plateaus* (Continuum, 2004). For helpful commentary on these difficult texts see Philip Goodchild, *Deleuze and Guattari: An Introduction to the Politics of Desire* (Sage, 1996).

16 See Camille Robcis, *Disalienation: Politics, Philosophy, and Radical Psychiatry in Postwar France* (Chicago University Press, 2021), 74–106.

17 For an astute analysis see Angela Woods, *The Sublime Object of Psychiatry: Schizophrenia in Clinical and Cultural Theory* (Oxford University Press, 2011), 145–61, in which Woods argues that 'Deleuze and Guattari's model of a revolutionary form of schizophrenia is doubly problematic: first because it cannot be defended against becoming "mere" pathology, and secondly because its political efficacy is dependent on, and I suggest limited by, its association with the sublime' (147).

18 See Frederic Jameson, *Postmodernism, or The Cultural Logic of Late Capitalism* (Duke University Press, 1990), 26–32. On Baudrillard see Woods, *Sublime Object*, 186–89; on schizophrenia and postmodernity in general, see 183–202.

19 For an overview see *Work, Psychiatry and Society, c.1750–2015*, ed. Waltraud Ernst (Manchester University Press, 2016).

20 For 'the coercive uses of psychology in UK government workfare programmes' see Lynne Friedli and Robert Stearn, 'Positive Affect as Coercive Strategy: Conditionality, Activation and the Role of Psychology in UK Government Workfare Programmes', *Medical Humanities* 41 (2015): 40–47.

21 For general overviews of the development of industrial psychology see Thompson, *Psychological Subjects*, 140–72 and *Historical Perspectives in Industrial and Organizational Psychology*, ed. Laura Koppes Bryan (Routledge, 2020). For specific applications see Maarten Derksen, 'Turning Men into Machines? Scientific Management, Industrial Psychology, and the "Human Factor"', *Journal of the History of the Behavioral Sciences* 50, no. 2 (2014): 148–65 and John C. Burnham, *Accident Prone: A History of Technology, Psychology, and Misfits of the Machine Age* (University of Chicago Press, 2009).

22 'Editorial Policy', *Human Relations* 1, no. 1 (1947): 1–2.

23 See Elizabeth Roberts-Pedersen, 'POWs into Citizens: Repatriation, Gender, and the Civilian Resettlement Units in Great Britain', in *Gender and Trauma Since 1900*, ed. Paula A. Michaels and Christina Twomey (Bloomsbury, 2021), 101–21.

24 Lester Coch and John R.P. French, 'Overcoming Resistance to Change', *Human Relations* 1, no. 4 (1947): 512 and 531.

25 Gerald M. Mahoney, 'Unidimensional Scales for The Measurement of Morale in an Industrial Situation', *Human Relations* 9, no. 1 (1956): 3–26.

26 J.M.M. Hill and E.L. Trist, 'A Consideration of Industrial Accidents as Means of Withdrawal from the Work Situation', *Human Relations* 6, no. 4 (1953): 357–80.

27 Clagett G. Smith and Arnold S. Tannenbaum, 'Organizational Control Structure: A Comparative Analysis', *Human Relations* 16, no. 4 (1963): 299–316.

28 Max Pagés, 'The Sociotherapy of the Enterprise: The Condition of Psycho-social Change in Industrial Concerns and the Role of the Social Psychologist as an Agent of Social Change', *Human Relations* 12, no. 4 (1959): 31–334.

29 On this point see Lucas Richert, *Break on Through: Radical Psychiatry and the American Counterculture* (The MIT Press, 2019), 19–25.

30 For an overview of the development of this discipline see Bruce E. Kaufman, *Managing the Human Factor: The Early Years of Human Resource Management in American Industry* (Cornell University Press, 2019), 36–54.

31 For an analysis of such training programs see Jessica Pykett and Byrony Enright, 'Geographies of Brain Culture: Optimism and Optimisation in Workplace Training Programmes', *Cultural Geographies* 23, no. 1 (2016): 51–68.

32 For a (pre-pandemic) overview see Anthony D. LaMontagne, et al., 'Workplace Mental Health: Developing an Integrated Intervention Approach', *BMC Psychiatry*, 14, no. 131 (2014).
33 'ILO Declaration on Fundamental Principles and Rights at Work', 2022 amendment: www.ilo.org/wcmsp5/groups/public/—ed_norm/—declaration/documents/normativeinstrument/wcms_716594.pdf.
34 Recent titles include Bev Aisbett, *The Book of Burn Out: What It Is, Why It Happens, Who Gets It, and How to Stop it Before It Stops You!* (Harper Collins, 2023); Anne Helen Petersen, *Can't Even: How Millennials Became the Burnout Generation* (Random House, 2022); Caroline Dooner, *Tired as F*ck: Burnout at the Hands of Diet, Self-Help, and Hustle Culture* (Harper Wave, 2022); Gordon Parker, Gabriela Tavella and Kerrie Eyers, *Burnout: A Guide to Identifying Burnout and Pathways to Recovery* (Allen & Unwin, 2021); Emily Nagoski and Amelia Nagoski, *Burnout: The Secret to Unlocking the Stress Cycle* (Ballantine Books, 2020).
35 Hannah Proctor, *Burnout: The Emotional Experience of Political Defeat* (Verso, 2024).
36 For an overview of understandings of 'stress' see David Cantor and Edmund Ramsden, 'Introduction', in *Stress, Shock, and Adaptation in the Twentieth Century*, ed. David Cantor and Edmund Ramsden (University of Rochester Press, 2014), 1–18.
37 Herbert J. Freudenberger, 'Staff Burn-Out', *Journal of Social Issues* 30, no. 1 (1974): 159–65; see also his paper of the following year, 'The Staff Burn-out Syndrome in Alternative Institutions', *Psychotherapy: Theory, Research & Practice* 12, no. 1 (1975): 73–82. The term may have been borrowed from drug-addicted clients to describe the effects of chronic drug use: see Matthew J. Hoffarth, 'The Making of Burnout: From Social Change to Self-awareness in the Postwar United States, 1970–82', *History of the Human Sciences* 30, no. 5 (2017): 35. For historical overviews from within the discipline see Flavio Muheim, 'Burnout: History of a Phenomenon', in *Burnout for Experts: Prevention in the Context of Living and Working*, ed. S. Bährer-Kohler (Springer, 2013), 37–46; Wilmar B. Schaufeli, 'Burnout: A Short Socio-Cultural History', in *Burnout, Fatigue, Exhaustion*, ed. S. Neckel, et al. (Palgrave, 2017), 105–27.
38 Freudenberger, 'Staff Burn-Out', 165.
39 Freudenberger, 'The Staff Burn-out Syndrome', 75.
40 Herbert J. Freudenberger with Geraldine Richelson, *Burn-out: The High Cost of High Achievement* (Doubleday, 1980); Christina Maslach, *Burnout, the Cost of Caring* (Prentice-Hall Press, 1986). See also the discussion in Hoffarth, 'The Making of Burnout', 30–45.
41 For examples of literature in this field see Thomas L. Schwenk and Katharine J. Gold, 'Physician Burnout—A Serious Symptom, But of What?', *JAMA* 320, no. 11 (280), 1109–10 and Daniel J. Madigan and Lisa E. Kim, 'Towards an Understanding of Teacher Attrition: A Meta-analysis of Burnout, Job Satisfaction, and Teachers' Intentions to Quit', *Teaching and Teacher Education* 104 (2021): 103425.
42 For an example from the United States see Grant L. Lin, et al., 'Resident and Fellow Unions: Collective Activism to Promote Well-being for Physicians in Training', *JAMA*, 328, no. 7 (2022): 619–20.
43 One study identified 142 separate definitions: see Lisa S. Rotenstein, et al., 'Prevalence of Burnout Among Physicians: A Systematic Review', *Journal of the American Medical Association* 320, no. 11 (2018): 1131–50.
44 For a discussion of the classification of burnout see Lindsey Nadon, et al., 'Should Burnout Be Conceptualized as a Mental Disorder?', *Behavioral Sciences* 12, no. 82 (2022), 1–1.
45 On the use of Thunberg's autism (among other tropes) see Emily D. Ryalls and Sharon R. Mazzarella, '"Famous, Beloved, Reviled, Respected, Feared, Celebrated": Media Construction of Greta Thunberg', *Communication, Culture and Critique* 14 (2021): 438–53.

46 See Glenn Albrecht, '"Solastalgia": A New Concept in Health and Identity', *PAN: Philosophy, Activism, Nature* 3 (2005): 49 and Glenn Albrecht, et al., 'Solastalgia: The Distress Caused by Environmental Change', *Australasian Psychiatry* 15, no. 1 (2007): S95–S98.
47 Glenn A. Albrecht, *Earth Emotions: New Words for a New World* (Cornell University Press, 2019).
48 See for example James H. Dunk, et al., 'Human Health on an Ailing Planet—Historical Perspectives on Our Future', *New England Journal of Medicine* 381 (2019): 778–82.
49 The consensus seems to be that the harms of social media can only be established as 'associational': for overviews see Betul Keles, et al., 'A Systematic Review: The Influence of Social Media on Depression, Anxiety and Psychological Distress in Adolescents', *International Journal of Adolescence and Youth* 25, no. 1 (2020): 79–93. See also Carol Vidal, et al., 'Social Media Use and Depression in Adolescents: A Scoping Review', *International Review of Psychiatry* 32, no. 3 (2020): 235.
50 On the question of what is eHealth/digital health see T. Shaw, et al., 'What Is eHealth (6)? Development of a Conceptual Model for eHealth: Qualitative Study with Key Informants', *Journal of Medical Internet Research* 19, no. 10 (2017): e324.
51 See P. Musiat and N. Tarrier, 'Collateral Outcomes in e-Mental Health: A Systematic Review of the Evidence for Added Benefits of Computerised Cognitive Behaviour Therapy Interventions for Mental Health', *Psychological Medicine* 44, no. 15 (2014): 3137–50.
52 Gerhard Andersson and Pim Cuijpers, 'Pros and Cons of Cognitive-Behavioural Therapy', *BJP* 193, no. 4 (2008): 270–71.
53 See for example R. Arjadi, et al., 'A Systematic Review of Online Interventions for Mental Health in Low and Middle Income Countries: A Neglected Field', *Global Mental Health* 14, no. 2 (2015): e12.
54 See for example Deborah Warr, et al., 'Hype, Evidence Gaps and Digital Divides: Telehealth Blind Spots in Rural Australia', *Health: An Interdisciplinary Journal for the Social Study of Health, Illness and Medicine* 27 (2023): 588–606.
55 See Rolfe Winkler, 'The Failed Promise of Online Mental-health Treatment', *Wall Street Journal* (19 December 2022), www.wsj.com/articles/the-failed-promise-of-online-mental-health-treatment-11671390353. For a very recent review of these and other apps, see Eunkyung Jo, et al., 'Exploring User Perspectives of and Ethical Experiences with Teletherapy Apps: Qualitative Analysis of User Reviews', *JMIR Mental Health* 10 (2023): e49684.
56 For helpful overviews of the direction of computational psychiatry see Quentin J.M. Huys, et al., 'Advances in the Computational Understanding of Mental Illness', *Neuropsychopharmacology Reviews* 46 (2021): 3–19; David Bennet, et al., 'The Two Cultures of Computational Psychiatry', *JAMA Psychiatry*, June 2019, 563; and Tobias U. Hauser, et al., 'The Promise of a Model-based Psychiatry: Building Computational Models of Mental Ill Health', *The Lancet: Digital Health* (October 2022).
57 P. Read Montague, et al., 'Computational Psychiatry', *Trends in Cognitive Sciences* 16 (2012), 72; for overviews of the contemporary state of the brain-as-computer debate see Giorgio Matassi, et al., 'Editorial: Current Thoughts on the Brain—Computer Analogy—All Metaphors Are Wrong, But Some Are Useful', *Frontiers in Ecology and Evolution* 11 (2023), 1–3; D.J. Kelty-Stephenson, et al., 'In Search for an Alternative to the Computer Metaphor of the Mind and Brain' *arXiv*, arXiv:2206.04603; and *The Routledge Handbook of the Computational Mind*, ed. Mark Sprevak and Matteo Colombo (Routledge, 2019). For an historical overview see Gerd Gigerenzer, *Adaptive Thinking: Rationality in the Real World* (Oxford University Press, 2002), 26–43.
58 Montague, 'Computational Psychiatry', 75.
59 See discussion in John Torous, et al., 'The Growing Field of Digital Psychiatry: Current Evidence and the Future of Apps, Social Media, Chatbots, and Virtual Reality', *World Psychiatry* 20, no. 3 (2021): 318–35.

60 Christian A. Webb, et al., 'Personalized Prediction of Antidepressant *v.* Placebo Response: Evidence from the EMBARC Study', *Psychological Medicine* 49 (2019): 1118–27.

61 For explanations of the formal thought disorder (FTD) thesis see Nancy C. Andreasen and William M. Grove, 'Thought, Language, and Communication in Schizophrenia: Diagnosis and Prognosis', *Schizophrenia Bulletin* 12 (1986): 348–59. For the means of demonstrating FTD in patients see Brita Elvevåg, et al., 'Quantifying Incoherence in Speech: An Automated Methodology and Novel Application to Schizophrenia', *Schizophrenia Research* 93 (2007): 304–16; Cheryl Mary Cocoran and Guillermo A. Cecchi, 'Using Language Processing and Speech Analysis for the Identification of Psychosis and Other Disorders', *Biological Psychiatry: Cognitive Neuroscience and Neuroimaging* 5 (2020): 770–79; and Isaac Franklin, et al., 'Theory-Driven Analysis of Natural Language Processing Measures of Thought Disorder Using Generative Language Modeling', *Biological Psychiatry: Cognitive Neuroscience and Neuroimaging* 8 (2023): P1013–23.

62 On this problem of prediction see Albert Rosen, 'Detection of Suicidal Patients: An Example of Some Limitations in the Prediction of Infrequent Events', *Journal of Consulting Psychology* 18, no. 6 (1954): 397–403.

63 For a general overview see Alban Lejeune, et al., 'Artificial Intelligence and Suicide Prevention: A Systematic Review', *European Psychiatry* 17, no. 16 (2022): 5929; for the use of emergency department datasets see Marie-Hélène Metzger, et al., 'Use of Emergency Department Electronic Medical Records for Automated Epidemiological Surveillance of Suicide Attempts: A French Pilot Study', *International Journal of Methods in Psychiatric Research* 26, no. 2 (2017): e1522 and Michael Sanderson, et al., 'Predicting Death by Suicide Following an Emergency Department Visit for Parasuicide with Administrative Health Care System Data and Machine Learning', *eClinicalMedicine* 20 (2020): 1–9.

64 Some of these issues are canvassed in the current Australian inquiry into veteran suicide: see Royal Commission into Defence and Veteran Suicide, *Interim Report* (11 August 2022), https://defenceveteransuicide.royalcommission.gov.au/publications/royal-commission-defence-and-veteran-suicide-interim-report.

65 See John F. McCarthy, et al., 'Predictive Modeling and Concentration of the Risk of Suicide: Implications for Preventive Interventions in the US Department of Veterans Affairs', *American Journal of Public Health* 105, no. 9 (2015): 1935–42 and John F. McCarthy, et al., 'Evaluation of the Recovery Engagement and Coordination for Health—Veterans Enhanced Treatment Suicide Risk Modelling Clinical Program in the Veterans Health Administration', *JAMA* 4, no. 10 (2021): 1–11.

66 See for example Sebastian Laacke, et al., 'Artificial Intelligence, Social Media and Depression. A New Concept of Health-Related Digital Autonomy', *The American Journal of Bioethics* 21, no. 7 (2021): 4–20. On the issue of gaps see Joshua August Skorburg and Phoebe Friesen, 'Mind the Gaps: Ethical and Epistemic Issues in the Digital Mental Health Response to Covid-19', *Hastings Center Report* (November–December 2021), which identifies four 'gaps': limited evidence as to the efficacy of 'newer digital mental health tools'; unequal or impeded access to digital tools (such as poor internet access or a lack of privacy; the inability of predictive tools to explain the phenomenon it predicts or to intervene effectively; and the potential for predictive models to put people in harm's way (such as police conducting wellness checks).

67 Mark A. Reger, et al., 'Patient Feedback on the Use of Predictive Analytics for Suicide Prevention', *Psychiatric Services* 72, no. 2 (2021): 129–35.

68 Trishan Panch, et al., 'Artificial Intelligence and Algorithmic Bias: Implications for Health Systems', *Journal of Global Health* 9, no. 2 (2019): 010318.

69 Lena Palaniyappan, 'More than a Biomarker: Could Language Be a Biosocial Marker of Psychosis?', *NPJ Schizophrenia* 42 (2021): 1–5.

70 Ellen E. Lee, et al., 'Artificial Intelligence for Mental Health Care: Clinical Applications, Barriers, Facilitators, and Artificial Wisdom', *Biological Psychiatry: Cognitive Neuroscience and Neuroimaging* 6, no. 9 (2021): 856–64.
71 Joseph Weizenbaum, 'ELIZA—A Computer Program for the Study of Natural Language Communication Between Man and Machine', *Communications of the ACM* 9, no. 1 (1966): 36–45.
72 On Rogers' therapeutic approach see Katja Guenther, '"Um, mm-h, Yeah": Carl Rogers, Phonographic Recordings, and the Making of Therapeutic Listening', *History of Psychology* 25, no. 3 (2022): 191–210.
73 For detailed overviews of Weizenbaum and his career see Simone Natale, 'The ELIZA Effect: Joseph Weizenbaum and the Emergence of Chatbots', in *Deceitful Media: Artificial Intelligence and Social Life after the Turing Test* (Oxford Academic, 2021), 60–65 and Elizabeth A. Wilson, *Affect and Artificial Intelligence* (University of Washington Press, 2010), 83–108.
74 Kenneth Mark Colby, James B. Watt and John P. Gilbert, 'A Computer Method of Psychotherapy: Preliminary Communication', *Journal of Nervous and Mental Disease* 142, no. 2 (1966): 148.
75 Colby, et al., 'A Computer Method of Psychotherapy', 150 and 152.
76 See Wilson, *Affect and Artificial Intelligence*, 99–100.
77 Joseph Weizenbaum, 'Computers as "Therapists"', *Science* 198, no. 4315 (1977): 354.
78 See Myron S. Denholtz and Edward Mann, 'Automated Treatment for Flight Phobia: A 3½-Year Follow-up', *American Journal of Psychiatry* 135, no. 11 (1978): 1340–43. The original study is Myron S. Denholtz and Edward T. Mann, 'Automated Audiovisual Treatment of Phobias Administered by Nonprofessionals', *Journal of Behaviour Therapy and Experimental Psychiatry* 6 (1975): 111–15.
79 See for example Johan Lundin, et al., 'Using 360-degree Videos for Virtual Reality Exposure in CBT for Panic Disorder with Agoraphobia: A Feasibility Study', *Behavioural and Cognitive Psychotherapy* 50, no. 2 (2021): 158–70.
80 Kenneth Mark Colby, 'Ethics of Computer-Assisted Psychotherapy', *Psychiatric Annals* 16, no. 7 (1986), 414–15.
81 Guy Laban, et al., 'Social Robots for Supporting Post-traumatic Stress Disorder Diagnosis and Treatment', *Frontiers in Psychiatry* 12 (2022): article 752874.
82 For an overview of research indicating that survey takers are more likely to disclose 'sensitive behaviours' when responding to computerised surveys see Timo Gnambs and Kai Kaspar, 'Disclosure of Sensitive Behaviours Across Self-administered Survey Modes: A Meta-analysis', *Behaviour Research Methods* 47 (2015): 1237–59.
83 See Gale M. Lucas, et al., 'Reporting Mental Health Symptoms: Breaking Down Barriers to Care with Virtual Human Interviewers', *Frontiers in Robotics and AI* 4 (2017): 1–9 and Gale M. Lucas, et al., 'It's Only a Computer: Virtual Humans Increase Willingness to Disclose', *Computers in Human Behaviour* 37 (2014): 94–100.
84 See Sherry Turkle, *The Second Self: Computers and the Human Spirit* (MIT Press, 2005); see also Wilson, 'Artificial Psychotherapy', 89–91.
85 Jerry Tang, et al., 'Semantic Reconstruction of Continuous Language from Non-invasive Brain Recordings', *Nature Neuroscience* 26 (2023): 858–66.
86 See for example 'AI Makes Non-invasive Mind-reading Possible by Turning Thoughts into Text', *The Guardian* (2 May 2023), www.theguardian.com/technology/2023/may/01/ai-makes-non-invasive-mind-reading-possible-by-turning-thoughts-into-text and 'This Machine Can Read Your Mind and Translate How You See the World', *BBC Science Focus* (2 May 2023), www.sciencefocus.com/news/this-machine-can-read-your-mind-and-translate-how-you-see-the-world.
87 For a recent description of one such device see Sean L. Metzger, et al., 'A High-performance Neuroprosthesis for Speech Decoding and Avatar Control', *Nature* 620

(2023): 1037–46. See also 'A Stroke Stole Her Ability to Speak at 30. A.I. Is Helping to Restore It Years Later', *New York Times* (23 August 2023), www.nytimes.com/2023/08/23/health/ai-stroke-speech-neuroscience.html.

88 For some of these functions (and a bit of boosterism) see Elena Sajno, et al., 'Machine Learning in Biosignals Processing for Mental Health: A Narrative Review', *Frontiers in Psychology* 13 (2022): 1–24.

89 Yang, 'Semantic Reconstruction', 862. For commentary on ethical issues see Stephen Rainey, et al., 'Brain Recording, Mind-reading, and Neurotechnology: Ethical Issues from Consumer Devices to Brain-based Speech Decoding', *Science and Engineering Ethics* 26, no. 4 (2020): 2295–11. Some of these issues are also canvassed in Nita A. Farahany, *The Battle for Your Brain: Defending the Right to Think Freely in the Age of Neurotechnology* (St. Martin's Press, 2023).

90 For some preliminary research on the ability to decipher dreams see T. Horikawa, et al., 'Neural Decoding of Visual Imagery During Sleep', *Science* 340, no. 6132 (2013): 639–42.

CONCLUSION

In this book, I have argued that a critical approach to the history of psychiatry and mental health positions them as dual endeavours—as clinical undertakings, but also as projects with distinct political effects. While the seeds of this clinical–political intersection were planted in the mid-nineteenth century, it began to bloom in the first decades of the twentieth century in response to the mental hygiene movement and the fallout from the First World War, and it flourished in the aftermath of the Second World War, which established psychiatry's usefulness in managing large-scale psychiatric casualties. By the early post-war period, mental health was an established concept and psychiatry an elevated specialty, promoted by both post-war governments and the World Health Organization (WHO) as integral to the reconstruction of liberal democratic norms and geopolitical stability. Over the ensuing decades, however, this overt political significance was increasingly obscured by a rising biological sensibility that reinscribed mental health and illness as the result of biomedical processes and refigured psychiatry and allied disciplines as biomedical ventures. This worldview was eventually formalised, though not without controversy, in the third edition of the *Diagnostic and Statistical Manual* (DSM-III), published in 1980. Yet this putative depoliticisation is belied by the continued political entanglements of psychiatry and mental health. Critical histories of mental health and psychiatry can help map this contested terrain, as well as describe both the circumstances and effects of its formation. In these concluding comments, I suggest some future directions framed around the themes explored in this book, as well as three broader areas of inquiry.

As discussed in Chapter 1, the asylum has been a central preoccupation for historians of psychiatry, prompting both close investigations of individual institutions, as well as more encompassing and controversial accounts seeking to explain its rise and fall in various national and international contexts. These efforts remain crucial

DOI: 10.4324/9780429351464-8

lines of inquiry, not least because the results demonstrate the variety between and even within institutions, as well as the continuities and discontinuities in local, regional, and national practices. Importantly, close attention to individual institutions can also disclose the way race, gender, sexuality, and other categories shaped the therapeutic approach of clinicians, the experience of patients, and the relationships between these interactions and the production of psychiatric knowledge. Yet expanding the view beyond traditional asylums and into other spaces that straddle the carceral and the putatively therapeutic–psychiatric wards of general hospitals, drug rehabilitation facilities, halfway houses, and group homes, as well as the prisons and nursing homes discussed in Chapter 1, would more accurately characterise the custodial responses to psychiatric distress, as well as deepen our understandings of the outcomes of deinstitutionalisation. Finally, listening for the voices of patients in such institutions and spaces, however fleeting and fragmentary, remains a central and urgent challenge for the discipline.

While Chapter 2 focused on the development of somatic and psychopharmaceutical therapies in the twentieth century and their relationship to the biomedicalisation of psychiatry and mental health, the study of 'psy' therapeutics in their entirety—from the 'blooding' practised by Monro at Bedlam to the re-emergence of psychedelics in the present—yields important insight into the relationship between psychiatric theory and therapeutic practice. This is not necessarily straightforward, as we have seen. On the one hand, the history of psychopharmacology suggests that the discovery of an effective therapy often prompted a post hoc theorising regarding the origins of the conditions it treated, exemplified by the various 'deficiency' hypothesises related to bipolar disorder (lithium), schizophrenia (dopamine), and depression (serotonin). Yet not all clinicians were interested in the causal mechanisms of the conditions they treated, regarding such inquiries as separate from immediate therapeutic concerns. More research into how these diverging attitudes translated into therapeutic approaches would go some way to reconstructing the patient experience of various clinical spaces, including those beyond the walls of the asylum, hospital, or general practitioner's office. It would also help illuminate the complex relationship between the development of various therapies and the evolution of psychiatric theory. Finally, continuing to historicise the evolution of 'neuro' discourses will also be decisive in conceptualising their relevance to past and current understandings of psychiatry and mental health.

Research into the relationship between psychiatry, mental health, and the state can also be expanded. While Chapter 3 highlights the emergence of public health and the mass warfare of the first half of the twentieth century as key factors in establishing these links, many other areas of intersection can benefit from historicisation–fiscal policy (health spending and scientific grant programs, for example), education policy, welfare policy, the criminal justice system, and the law more broadly, including the attitude towards civil liberties, bodily autonomy, and consent, to name just a few. The use of mental health and psychiatry by repressive regimes (or by notionally democratic governments for repressive ends) also warrants continued attention. Beyond extreme examples like Nazi Germany and the Soviet Union, how have governments used concepts associated with psychiatry and mental health to identify, manage, or otherwise persecute their opponents or other undesirable individuals or communities? How have clinicians responded to these actions? And to what extent can we recover the experience of the individuals targeted by such programs? Thinking historically about this instrumentalisation demonstrates the diffusion of clinical concepts beyond strictly clinical spaces.

Tensions between the universal and the particular in the history of psychiatry and mental health will continue to be a fruitful avenue of inquiry. Chapter 4 traces the links between colonial psychiatry, the mental health agenda of the early World Health Organization, the anti-colonial and Indigenous psychiatries that emerged in the decades after the Second World War, and the evolution of global mental health as a concern of international health agencies. All four instances indicate the political stakes of designating psychiatric conditions as either universal or culturally (and, in colonial contexts, racially) specific. Beyond colonial settings, historians continue to investigate the ways psychiatry and mental health were racialised in national contexts, such as the United States and South Africa—inquiries that can be expanded to other nations across a variety of timescales.[1] Moreover, these questions can be generalised. In what other cases have the universal and the particular been in a contest in the formation of psychiatric diagnoses, what have been the outcomes of this contest, and how has this been mobilised for political ends? In addition to race, continuing to trace the operation of gender and class in psychiatric theorising and practice offers an important means of understanding the way psychiatric diagnoses can promulgate hierarchies that are politically salient.

Questions of race and gender were also at issue in Chapter 5, which considered dissent within the American Psychiatric Association (APA) during the 1960s and 1970s over the psychoanalytic precepts that shaped American psychiatry in the decades after the Second World War, as well as the challenge to psychiatric authority presented by mad activists from this period onwards. While this focus on the United States reflects the influence of the APA and its *Diagnostic and Statistical Manual* on Anglophone psychiatry during this period, the central themes of authority and dissent can be profitably traced beyond the United States—an exercise that would also contextualise the impact of American psychiatry on clinical theory and practice elsewhere. Questions might include how psychiatric authority was formed in different contexts and in what ways was it distinctive to certain periods, national contexts, and institutions; how both clinicians and patients responded to such authority; how the guardians of such authority have responded to discontent; how dissent manifested in different periods and in different venues (institutions, professional societies, the medical press, and so on); and how such disagreements informed both psychiatric theory and practice.

Finally, historical relationships between a prevailing economic order and ideas about mental health can also be explored in greater depth than the account of capitalist psychopolitics offered in Chapter 6. For example, how have different capitalist economies at different times been understood to interact with individual and collective psyches? More concretely, how have these capitalist economies instrumentalised and monetised the practice of psychiatry and the concept of mental health? In what other ways has work been psychiatrised, and what other avenues exist for the marketisation of digital therapies? Finally, as we saw in Chapter 3, scholars working on the history of psychiatry in the Soviet Union have emphasised not just the way psychiatry was used against opponents of the regime, but also the expectation that theories about the mechanisms causing psychiatric distress would reflect doctrinal orthodoxy. To what extent were these tendencies evident in other socialist states, and how did this affect the experience of patients and clinicians? In addition, is it possible to characterise socialism as advocating a species of psychopolitics—either in opposition to an imagined capitalist psychopolitics or as a feature of these economic arrangements—and if so, what are its distinguishing features? Critically examining the effects of economic arrangements on the practice of psychiatry, as well as the theorisation of relationships between the economic order and the constitution of the psyche, offers ways of understanding the resilience but also contingency of these arrangements.

Three additional issues strike me as particularly important and worthy of further thought. The first is the way psychiatry and mental health are capable not just of politicisation but of generating distinctive modes of politics—arrangements that we may refer to generally as psychopolitics but more specifically as, for example, neuro-politics or trauma politics. Here, the history of trauma theory and its reception offers a particularly resonant example of the way a psychiatric concept might achieve significant political status. As we saw in Chapter 3, it was the political claims of anti-war Vietnam veterans and their clinicians, drawing on theories developed to explain the persisting symptoms of Holocaust survivors, that helped transform Post Vietnam Syndrome into post-traumatic stress disorder. Once installed in DSM-III, the diagnosis was a mechanism to make the suffering of several kinds of victims legible and legitimate: veterans and other victims of war; victims of rape, assault, and other forms of violence; and survivors of life-threatening accidents, injuries, illnesses, and natural disasters. Soon, however, the category expanded to include not just direct victims but traumatised witnesses, such as first responders. Associated forms of trauma were also hypothesised, such as intergenerational and collective trauma. And, as scholars like Ruth Leys have shown, trauma and PTSD soon transcended the clinical realm, were installed in culture, and instrumentalised in the academy.[2] In addition, as Didier Fassin and Richard Rechtman argued in an important book, trauma gave certain groups the status of legitimate victims.[3] Yet this political visibility comes with caveats. It can be bestowed from afar in a hegemonic gesture (in Fassin and Rechtmann's example, in disaster regions of the Global South). It can be used to promote or justify violence. And not everyone qualifies as a suitable victim because victim status remains a political question. In the early literature on PSTD, for example, Black veterans appear to have been diagnosed with the condition less frequently than white veterans perhaps because, as one study suggested, '[t]he [B]lack male presenting as distrustful, angry, and with a combat history has considerable potential to alarm white clinicians, potentiating diagnostic error and treatment failure.'[4] Thus, though PTSD has in theory put more clinical emphasis on the traumatic event itself, it is still possible to extend or deny the diagnosis to certain individuals or groups. Tracing the implications of the various forms of trauma politics thus remains an important task.

This leads to a second encompassing issue: the interactions between psychiatry and marginalised communities, both historically and in the present. While a critical approach to the history of psychiatry and mental health indicates that psychiatry has at times been used against the powerful, it is less clear whether it has helped or hindered the pursuit of equity and justice—either conceptually, or in material terms. While this inheres in many contexts, it is particularly relevant in terms of the Global North/South divide. An increasingly globalised psychiatry not only raises the problematic and perhaps irresolvable tension between the universal and the particular, but asks questions about equity of access to research (including research design) and treatment. Critics of global mental health argue that it is not sufficient to import Western notions of mental health into the Global South and that a better approach is to trouble Western certainties by including clinicians and patients from the Global South as equal partners in research efforts. Similarly, therapeutics normalised in Western contexts may be difficult to apply elsewhere; these attempts could be the subject of further historical research. In the present day, global flows of psychopharmaceuticals are one important avenue for assessing these effects.

The third and final point returns to the problem of 'kinds' canvassed in the Introduction and evident throughout this book—the fact that there is no consensus on both what mental illness 'is' or, indeed, whether this lack of certainty matters. An increasing appreciation of the complexity of the brain and the corresponding brain–body system will likely make this problem of kinds a persistent issue, as researchers strive to show the neurological correlates of symptoms and behaviours as a way to make mental illness unimpeachably 'real.' For that reason, a critical approach to mental health requires taking seriously the influence of neuroscience and biomedicine on the way that mental health is conceptualised. Reframing biomedical factors as *biocultural* appears a particularly urgent task as AI capabilities increase and shape the nature of inquiries into psychiatric distress. Thinking critically about kinds also impels attention to questions of degree—that is, how to maintain distinctions in severity; to distinguish between, for example, a patient suffering from schizophrenia and a patient suffering from social anxiety; distinctions that guide the allocation of resources and attention. For this reason, putting all forms of mental disorder under the umbrella of 'mental health' is not only inaccurate but also unjust.

As I have suggested in this book, such imprecision is central to, and perhaps constitutive of, both psychiatry as a discipline and the notion of mental health it sustains. Indeed, my sense is that the euphemistic, ambiguous quality of 'mental health' identified by Huw Green and cited in the Introduction is precisely what explains the concept's durability and continued expansion into much of contemporary life. By signifying both illness and health, mental health exemplifies the flexibility and adaptability that the sum of its discourses presents as personal virtues and therapeutic aims. In this way, it absorbs and reproduces some of the central paradoxes of psychiatry, whose own expansion from the asylum to mainstream medicine charts a similar path from niche concern to general application, from florid madness to the infinite varieties of human distress. For that reason, to the extent that psychiatry and mental health have made human distress their object, their longevity is guaranteed, because the problem they confront is probably insoluble. If that is the case, then history suggests that what we call mental illness is both a test of our humanity and also a confirmation of it. If we are to really move past stigma and not just engage in 'benevolent othering,' then hard truths—about the reality of mental illness, but also about the limits of our knowledge about such conditions—must not be stigmatising.[5] Pursuing critical histories of psychiatry and mental health not only contextualises present challenges but poses possibilities for alternative futures.

Notes

1 See for example Wendy Gonaver, *The Peculiar Institution and the Making of Modern Psychiatry, 1840–1880* (University of North Carolina Press, 2018), and Tiffany Fawn Jones, *Psychiatry, Mental Institutions, and the Mad in Apartheid South Africa* (Routledge, 2012).

2 Ruth Leys, *Trauma: A Genealogy* (University of Chicago Press, 2000).

3 Didier Fassin and Richard Rechtmann, *The Empire of Trauma: An Inquiry into the Condition of Victimhood*, trans. Rachel Gomme (Princeton University Press, 2009).

4 Irving M. Allen, 'Posttraumatic Stress Disorder Among Black Vietnam Veterans', *Psychiatric Services* 37 (1986): 57.

5 See for example Flick Grey, 'Benevolent Othering: Speaking Positively about Mental Health Service Users', *Philosophy, Psychiatry & Psychology* 23 (2016): 241–51.

REFERENCES

Aalbers, Dan, 'The Hoffman Report in Historical Context: A Study in Denial', *History of the Human Sciences* 35, no. 5 (2022): 27.

Abi-Rached, Joelle M., *'Asfūriyyeh: A History of Madness, Modernity, and War in the Middle East*. The MIT Press, 2020.

Adam, John, et al., 'Perspectives on Erving Goffman's "Asylums" Fifty Years On', *Medicine, Health Care, and Philosophy* 16 (2013): 605–13.

Adler-Bolton, Beatrice, and Artie Vierkant, *Health Communism*. Verso, 2022.

'Admitting Committee', in Neville T. Yeomans Papers, 1960–1971, State Library of New South Wales, MLMSS. 2416/2, Papers re Fraser House, 1960–1967.

Adorno, Theodor W., *The Authoritarian Personality*. Harper & Row, 1950.

Aho, Tanja, Liat Ben-Moshe and Leon J. Hilton, 'Mad Futures: Affect/Theory/Violence', *American Quarterly* 69, no. 2 (2017): 291–302.

Aisbett, Bev, *The Book of Burn Out: What It Is, Why It Happens, Who Gets It, and How to Stop it Before It Stops You*! Harper Collins, 2023.

Albrecht, Glenn A., *Earth Emotions: New Words for a New World*. Cornell University Press, 2019.

Albrecht, Glenn A., '"Solastaglia": A New Concept in Health and Identity', *PAN: Philosophy, Activism, Nature* 3 (2005): 49.

Albrecht, Glenn A., et al., 'Solastalgia: The Distress Caused by Environmental Change', *Australasian Psychiatry* 15, no. 1 (2007): S95–S98.

Allen, Irving M., 'Posttraumatic Stress Disorder Among Black Vietnam Veterans', *Psychiatric Services* 37 (1986): 55–61.

Allen, J.R., and L.J. West, 'Flight from Violence: Hippies and the Green Rebellion', *American Journal of Psychiatry* 125, no. 3 (1968): 364–70.

'AI Makes Non-invasive Mind-reading Possible by Turning Thoughts into Text', *The Guardian*, 2 May 2023, www.theguardian.com/technology/2023/may/01/ai-makes-non-invasive-mind-reading-possible-by-turning-thoughts-into-text.

Alphin, Caroline, and François Debrix, 'Biopolitics in the "Psychic Realm": Han, Foucault and Neoliberal Psychopolitics', *Philosophy & Social Criticism* 49, no. 4 (2021): 477–91.

Amrith, Sunil S., *Decolonising International Health: India and Southeast Asia, 1930–65*. Palgrave, 2006.

Anderson, David, 'British Abuse and Torture in Kenya's Counter-insurgency, 1952–1960', *Small Wars and Insurgencies* 23, no. 4–5 (2012): 700–19.

Anderson, Warwick, 'The Trespass Speaks: White Masculinity and Colonial Breakdown', *American Historical Review* 102, no. 5 (1997): 1343–70.

Anderson, Warwick, Deborah Jenson, and Richard C. Keller, eds., *Unconscious Dominions: Psychoanalysis, Colonial Trauma, and Global Sovereignties*. Duke University Press, 2011.

Andersson, Gerhard, and Pim Cuijpers, 'Pros and Cons of Cognitive-Behavioural Therapy', *British Journal of Psychiatry* 193, no. 4 (2008): 270–71.

Andreasen, Nancy C., and William M. Grove, 'Thought, Language, and Communication in Schizophrenia: Diagnosis and Prognosis', *Schizophrenia Bulletin* 12 (1986): 348–59.

Andrews, Jonathan, and Anne Digby, eds., *Sex and Seclusion, Class and Custody: Gender and Class in the History of British and Irish Psychiatry*. Rodopi, 2004.

Andrews, Jonathan, and Andrew Scull, *Customers and Patrons of the Mad-Trade: The Management of Lunacy in Eighteenth-Century London*. University of California Press, 2003.

Andrews, Jonathan, and Andrew Scull, *Undertaker of the Mind: John Monro and Mad-doctoring in Eighteenth-century England*. University of California Press, 2001.

Angelini, Alberto, 'History of the Unconscious in Soviet Russia: From Its Origins to the Fall of the Soviet Union', *International Journal of Psychoanalysis* 89 (2008): 369–88.

Antić, Ana, 'Decolonizing Madness? Transcultural Psychiatry, International Order and Birth of a "Global Psyche" in the Aftermath of the Second World War', *Journal of Global History* 17 (2022): 21–22.

Antić, Ana, *Non-aligned Psychiatry in the Cold War: Revolution, Emancipation and Reimagining the Human Psyche*. Palgrave, 2021.

Appignanesi, Lisa, and John Forrester, *Freud's Women*. Virago Press, 1992.

Apple, Rima D., *Perfect Motherhood: Science and Childrearing in America*. Rutgers University Press, 2006.

Arias, Daniel et al., 'Quantiyfing the Global Burden of Mental Disorders and Their Economic Value', *eClinicalMedicine* 54 (2022): 101675.

Arjadi, R., et al., 'A Systematic Review of Online Interventions for Mental Health in Low and Middle Income Countries: A Neglected Field', *Global Mental Health* 14, no. 2 (2015): e12.

Arthur, R.J., 'Hospital Ship Psychiatry in a War Zone', *American Journal of Psychiatry* 124, no. 3 (1967): 281–86.

Atkinson, R.M., et al., 'Assessment of Viet Nam Veterans for Posttraumatic Stress Disorder in Veterans Administration Disability Claims', *American Journal of Psychiatry* 139, no. 9 (1982): 1118–21.

Australian Medical Association, 'AMA Submission to Pharmaceutical Benefits Advisory Committee—Restricted Prescription of Antipsychotics in Residential Aged Care', 20 October 2021, www.ama.com.au/articles/ama-submission-pbac-restricted-prescription-antipsychotics-residential-aged-care.

Australian Medical Association, 'AMA Submission to the Royal Commission into Aged Care Quality and Safety', www.ama.com.au/sites/default/files/documents/AMA_submission_to_the_Royal_Commission_into_Aged_Care_Quality_and_Safety_FINAL.pdf.

Australian Psychological Society, 'The APS Apology to Aboriginal and Torres Strait Islander People', *Australian Psychological Society*, 2017, https://psychology.org.au/community/reconciliation-and-the-aps/aps-apology.

Australian Psychology Accreditation Council, 'Accreditation Standards for Psychology Programs', 1 January 2019, https://apac.au/education-providers/standards/.

Ayo, Nike, 'Understanding Health Promotion in a Neoliberal Climate and the Making of Health Conscious Citizens', *Critical Public Health* 22, no. 1 (2012): 99–105.

Bacopoulos-Viau, Alexandra, and Aude Fauvel, 'The Patient's Turn: Roy Porter and Psychiatry's Tales, Thirty Years On', *Medical History* 60, no. 1 (2016): 1–18.

Baggally, A.R., 'Myths of Mau Mau Expanded: Rehabilitation in Kenya's Detention Camps, 1954–60', *Journal of Eastern African Studies* 5, no. 3 (2011): 553–78.

Baistow, K., 'Problems of Powerlessness: Psychological Explanations of Social Inequality and Civil Unrest in Postwar America', *History of the Human Sciences* 13, no. 3 (2000): 95–116.

Bar-Haim, Shual, *The Maternalists: Psychoanalysis, Motherhood, and the British Welfare State*. University of Philadelphia Press, 2021.

Barham, Peter, *Forgotten Lunatics of the Great War*. Yale University Press, 2007.

Barham, Peter, 'Foucault and the Psychiatric Practitioner', *History of the Human Sciences* 3, no. 3 (1990): 328.

Barrows, Howard S., 'Pseudopatients', *British Medical Journal* (15 March 1975): 625–26.

Barrows, Howard S., 'Simulated Patients in Medical Teaching', *Canadian Medical Association Journal* 98, no. 14 (1968): 674–76.

Bartova, Lucie, et al., 'Reply to: "The Serotonin Theory of Depression: A Systematic Umbrella Review of the Evidence"', *Molecular Psychiatry* 28, no. 8 (2022): 3153–54.

Bashford, Alison, *Imperial Hygiene: A Critical History of Colonialism, Nationalism and Public Health*. Palgrave Macmillan, 2003.

Bashford, Alison, and Philippa Levine, 'Introduction: Eugenics and the Modern World', in *The Oxford Handbook of the History of Eugenics*, ed. Alison Bashford and Philippa Levine. Oxford University Press, 2010, pp. 1–4.

Basso, Elisabetta, *Young Foucault: The Lille Manuscripts on Psychopathology, Phenomenology, and Anthropology, 1952–1955*. Columbia University Press, 2022.

Baumeister, Alan A., 'The Chlorpromazine Enigma', *Journal of the History of the Neurosciences* 22 (2013): 14–29.

Beard, George, 'Neurasthenia, or Nervous Exhaustion', *Boston Medical and Surgical Journal*, (29 April 1869): 217–21.

Beck, Aaron, 'Cognitive Therapy: Nature and Relation to Behavior Therapy', *Behavior Therapy* 1, no. 2 (1970): 184–200.

Beers, Clifford, *A Mind That Found Itself*. Longmans, Green, and Co, 1908.

Beliaeva, Anastasia, 'Creating the New Soviet Man: The Case of Neurasthenia', *Social History of Medicine* 35, no. 5 (2022): 927–45.

Belknap, Ivan, *Human Problems of a State Mental Hospital*. McGraw-Hill, 1956.

Benedict, Susan, and Tessa Chelouche, 'Meseritz-Obrawalde: A "Wild Euthanasia" Hospital of Nazi Germany', *History of Psychiatry* 19, no. 1 (2008): 68–76.

Bennet, David, et al., 'The Two Cultures of Computational Psychiatry', *Journal of the American Medical Association Psychiatry* (June 2019): 563.

Bennett, Huw, *Fighting the Mau Mau: The British Army and Counter-Insurgency in the Kenya Emergency*. Cambridge University Press, 2012.

Bennett, Huw, 'The Mau Mau Emergency as Part of the British Army's Post-War Counter-Insurgency Experience', *Defence & Security Analysis* 23 (2007): 143–63.

Berco, Cristian, 'Perception and the Mulatto Body in Inquisitorial Spain: A Neurohistory', *Past & Present* 231 (2016): 33–60.

Beresford, Peter, 'Introduction', in *The Routledge International Handbook of Mad Studies*, ed. Peter Beresford and Jasna Russo. Routledge, 2021, p. 1.

Bergenheim, Sophy, et al., eds., *Conceptualising Public Health: Historical and Contemporary Struggles Over Key Concepts*. Routledge, 2018, pp. 1–17.

Bergner, G., 'Black Children, White Preference: *Brown v. Board*, the Doll Test, and the Politics of Self-Esteem', *American Quarterly* 61, no. 2 (2009): 299–332.

Berman, Bruce, and John Lonsdale, 'Louis Leakey's Mau Mau: A Study in the Politics of Knowledge', *History and Anthropology* 5, no. 2 (1991): 143–204.

Berrios, G.E., 'The Scientific Origins of Electroconvulsive Therapy: A Conceptual History', *History of Psychiatry* viii (1997): 105–19.

Bérubé, Allan, *Coming Out Under Fire: The History of Gay Men and Women in World War II*. 2nd ed. University of North Carolina Press, 2010.

Bieber, Irving, 'Homosexual Dynamics in Psychiatric Crisis', *American Journal of Psychiatry* 128, no. 10 (1972): 1268–72.

Bieber, Irving, 'Homosexuality—An Adaptive Consequence of Disorder in Psychosexual Development' in R.J. Stoller et al., 'A Symposium: Should Homosexuality Be in the APA Nomenclature?', *American Journal of Psychiatry* 130, no. 11 (1973): 1207–16.
Blain, Daniel, 'Some Essentials in National Mental Health Planning', *BMC* (November 1946): 180–81.
Blayney, Steffan, 'Activist Sources and the Survivor Movement', in *Sources in the History of Psychiatry, from 1800 to the Present*, ed. Chris Millard and Jennifer Wallis. Routledge, 2022.
Bock, Cornelius, *Brainwaves: A Cultural History of Electroencephalography*, trans. Ann M. Hentschel. Routledge, 2018.
Boddice, Rob, *A History of Feelings*. Reaktion, 2019.
Boddice, Rob, and Daniel Lord Smail, 'Neurohistory', in *Debating New Approaches to History*, ed. Marek Tamm and Peter Burke. Bloomsbury Academic, 2018.
Boettcher, Lillian B., and Sarah T. Menacho, 'The Early Argument for Prefrontal Leucotomy: The Collision of Frontal Lobe Theory and Psychosurgery at the 1935 International Neurological Congress in London', *Neurological Focus* 43, no. 3 (2017): 1–7.
Bogowicz, Paul, et al., 'Trends and Variation in Antidepressant Prescribing in English Primary Care: A Retrospective Longitudinal Study', *BJGP Open* 5, no. 4 (2021).
Borch-Jacobsen, Mikkel, and Sonu Shamdasani, *The Freud Files: An Inquiry into the History of Psychoanalysis*. Cambridge University Press, 2011.
Bothwell, Laura E., and Scott H. Podolsky, 'The Emergence of the Randomized, Controlled Trial', *The New England Journal of Medicine* 375 (2016): 501–04.
Bowman, Karl M., and Bernice Engle, 'A Psychiatric Evaluation of Laws of Homosexuality', *American Journal of Psychiatry* 112, no. 8 (1956): 577–83.
Braslow, Joel T., 'The Influence of a Biological Therapy on Physicians' Narratives and Interrogations: The Case of General Paralysis of the Insane and Malaria Fever Therapy, 1910–1950', *Bulletin of the History of Medicine* 70, no. 4 (1996): 577–608.
Braslow, Joel T., *Mental Ills and Bodily Cures: Psychiatric Treatment in the First Half of the Twentieth Century*. University of California Press, 1997.
Brickman, H.R., 'The Psychedelic "Hip Scene": Return of the Death Instinct', *American Journal of Psychiatry* 125, no. 6 (1968): 78–84.
Brock, Laurence, 'Towards a Unified Mental Health Service', *Mental Welfare* 20, no. 4 (1939): 93–97.
Brody, D.J., and Q. Gu, 'Antidepressant Use Among Adults: United States, 2015–2018', *NCHS Data Brief No. 377*. National Center for Health Statistics, 2020.
Brown, Michael, 'Rethinking Early Nineteenth Century Asylum Reform', *The Historical Journal* 49, no. 2 (2006): 425–52.
Brown, Wendy, *Undoing the Demos: Neoliberalism's Stealth Revolution*. Zone Books, 2015.
Bruce-Lockhart, Katherine, '"Unsound" Minds and Broken Bodies: The Detention of "Hardcore" Mau Mau Women at Kamiti and Gitamaya Detention Camps in Kenya, 1954–1960', *Journal of Eastern African Studies* 8, no. 4 (2014): 590–608.
Bryant, Michael S., *Confronting the 'Good Death': Nazi Euthanasia on Trial, 1945–1953*. University Press of Colorado, 2005.
Buchanan, Roderick David, 'Review of The Great Pretender: The Undercover Mission That Changed Our Understanding of Madness', *Journal of the History of the Behavioural Sciences* 56, no. 1 (2020): 53.
Buckman, J., 'Social and Medical Aspects of Illicit Use of LSD', *International Journal of Social Psychiatry* 17, no. 3 (1971): 163–76.
Bueltzingsloewen, Isabelle Von, 'Starvation in French Asylums During the German Occupation (1940–1945): Methodological Issues in a Comparative Historical Investigation', in *Transnational Psychiatries: Social and Cultural Histories of Psychiatry in Comparative Perspective c.1800–2000*, ed. Waltraud Ernst and Thomas Mueller. Cambridge Scholars Publishing, 2010, pp. 229–43.
Buhle, Mari Jo, 'Feminists versus Freud', in *Feminism and Its Discontents: A Century of Struggle with Psychoanalysis*. Harvard University Press, 1998, pp. 206–39.

Buklijas, Tatjana, 'The Laboratory and the Asylum: Francis Walker Mott and the Pathological Laboratory at London County Council Lunatic Asylum, Claybury, Essex (1895–1916)', *History of Psychiatry* 28, no. 3 (2017): 311–25.

Burman, Jeremy Trevelyan, 'History from Within? Contextualising the New Neurohistory and Seeking Its Methods', *History of Psychology* 15 (2012): 84–99.

Burnham, John C., *Accident Prone: A History of Technology, Psychology, and Misfits of the Machine Age*. University of Chicago Press, 2009.

Burrett, Tina, and Jeff Kingston, eds., *Routledge Handbook of Trauma in East Asia*. Routledge, 2023.

Burrows, V., and B. Berney, 'Creating Equal Health Opportunity: How the Medical Civil Rights Movement and the Johnson Administration Desegregated US Hospitals', *Journal of American History* 105, no. 4 (2019): 885–91.

Burton, Mark, and Raquel Guzzo, 'Liberation Psychology: Origins and Development', in *Liberation Psychology: Theory, Method, Practice, and Social Justice*, ed. L. Comas-Díaz and E. Torres Rivera. American Psychological Association, 2020, pp. 17–40.

Byrne, Gerard J., 'Prescribing Psychotropic Medications in Residential Aged Care Facilities', *Medical Journal of Australia* 212, no. 7 (2020): 304–05.

Cade, J.F., 'Lithium Salts in the Treatment of Psychotic Excitement', *Medical Journal of Australia* 2, no. 10 (1949): 349–52.

Cahalan, Susannah, *The Great Pretender: The Undercover Mission that Changed Our Understanding of Madness*. Grand Central, 2019.

Canaday, Margot, *The Straight State: Sexuality and Citizenship in Twentieth Century America*. Princeton University Press, 2009.

Cantor, David, and Edmund Ramsden, 'Introduction', in *Stress, Shock, and Adaptation in the Twentieth Century*, ed. David Cantor and Edmund Ramsden. University of Rochester Press, 2014, pp. 1–18.

Caplan, Gerald, *An Approach to Community Mental Health*. Grune and Stratton, 1961.

Capps, Donald, 'Mental Illness, Religion, and the Rational Mind: The Case of Clifford W. Beers', *Mental Health, Religion & Culture* 12, no. 2 (2009): 157–74.

Carothers, J.C., *The African Mind in Health and Disease: A Study in Ethnopsychiatry*. World Health Organization, 1953.

Carothers, J.C., 'Frontal Lobe Function and the African', *Journal of Mental Science* 97, no. 406 (1951): 12.

Carothers, J.C., *The Psychology of Mau Mau*. The Government Printer, Nairobi, 1955.

Carpenter Jr, W.T., N.R. Tamarkin, and D.E. Raskin, 'Emergency Psychiatric Treatment During a Mass Rally: The March on Washington', *American Journal of Psychiatry* 127, no. 10 (1971): 1327–32.

Carrier, Felix, et al., 'Ethical Challenges in Developing Drugs for Psychiatric Disorders', *Progress in Neurobiology* 152 (2017): 58–69.

Caudill, William, et al., 'Social Structure and Interaction Processes on a Psychiatric Ward', *American Journal of Orthopsychiatry* 22 (1952): 315.

Chaney, Sarah, 'No "Sane" Person Would Have Any Idea': Patients' Involvement in Late Nineteenth-century British Asylum Psychiatry', *Medical History* 60, no. 1 (2016): 37–53.

Chapman, Adrian, 'Dwelling in Strangeness: Accounts of the Kingsley Hall Community, London (1965–1970), Established by R. D. Laing', *Journal of Medical Humanities* 42 (2021): 471–94.

Chappel, J.N., and R.S. Daniels, 'Home Visiting in a Black Urban Ghetto', *American Journal of Psychiatry* 126, no. 10 (1970): 1455–60.

Char, Jerome, 'Drug Abuse in Viet Nam', *American Journal of Psychiatry* 129, no. 4 (1972): 463–65.

Charland, Louis, 'Benevolent Theory: Moral Treatment at the York Retreat', *History of Psychiatry* 18, no. 1 (2007): 61–80.

Chase-Levenson, Alex, *The Yellow Flag: Quarantine and the British Mediterranean World, 1780–1860*. Cambridge University Press, 2020.

Chesher, G.B., 'Pseudopatients and Evaluation of Medical Practice', *Medical Journal of Australia* (26 October 1974): 643.
Chesler, Phyllis, *Women and Madness*. Avon, 1972.
Chessick, R.D., 'Review: Morton Levitt and Ben Rubenstein: *The Student Revolt: Totem and Taboo Revisited*', *American Journal of Psychotherapy* 25, no. 3 (1971): 493.
Cheyne, George, *The English Malady (1773)*. Routledge, 1991.
Chisholm, George Brock, 'Social Responsibility', *Science* 109, no. 2820 (1949): 27–43.
Ciofal, Nuria, et al., 'Indigenous Community Psychologies, Decolonisation, and Radical Imagination Within Ecologies of Knowledges', *American Journal of Community Psychology* 69, no. 3–4 (2022): 283–93.
Clark, Alfred W., and Neville T. Yeomans, *Fraser House: Theory, Practice, and Evaluation of a Therapeutic Community*. Springer, 1969.
Clark, Eileen, 'Lessons from the Past: Family Involvement in Patient Admission and Discharge, Beechworth Lunatic Asylum, 1900–1912', *International Journal of Mental Health Nursing* 27, no. 1 (2018): 320–28.
Clark, K.B., 'As Old as Human Cruelty', *The New York Times*, 22 September 1968: 373.
Clark, K.B., *Dark Ghetto: Dilemmas of Social Power*. Harper and Row, 1965.
Clark, Yvonne, and Tanja Hirvonen, 'Decolonising Australian Psychology: The Influence of Aboriginal Psychologists', in *Decolonial Enactments in Community Psychology*, ed. Shose Kessi, Shahnaaz Suffla and Mohamed Seedat. Springer Nature, 2021, pp. 213–33.
Clarke, Liam, 'The Opening of Doors in British Mental Hospitals in the 1950s', *History of Psychiatry* 4, no. 16 (1993): 527–51.
Cobb, Matthew, *The Idea of the Brain: A History*. Basic Books, 2021.
Coch, Lester, and John R.P. French, 'Overcoming Resistance to Change', *Human Relations* 1, no. 4 (1947): 512–31.
Cocks, Geoffrey, *Psychotherapy in the Third Reich: The Göring Institute*. Transaction Publishers, 1997.
Cocoran, Cheryl Mary, and Guillermo A. Cecchi, 'Using Language Processing and Speech Analysis for the Identification of Psychosis and Other Disorders', *Biological Psychiatry: Cognitive Neuroscience and Neuroimaging* 5 (2020): 770–79.
Cohen, Bruce M.Z., *Psychiatric Hegemony: A Marxist Theory of Mental Illness*. Palgrave, 2016.
Cohen, Irvin M., 'Complications of Chlorpromazine Therapy', *American Journal of Psychiatry* 113, no. 2 (1956): 115–21.
Colbach, E.M., and M.D. Parrish, 'Army Mental Health Activities in Vietnam: 1965–1970', *Bulletin of the Menninger Clinic* 34, no. 6 (1970): 333–42.
Colby, Kenneth Mark, 'A Computer Method of Psychotherapy', *Journal of Nervous and Mental Disease* 142, no. 2 (1966): 148–52.
Colby, Kenneth Mark, 'Ethics of Computer-Assisted Psychotherapy', *Psychiatric Annals* 16, no. 7 (1986): 414–15.
Colby, Kenneth Mark, 'Journal of Mental Science. XCVII, 1951: Frontal Lobe Function and the African. J.C. Carothers. Pp. 12–48', *The Psychoanalytic Quarterly* 21 (1952): 594–95.
Colby, Kenneth Mark, James B. Watt and John P. Gilbert, 'A Computer Method of Psychotherapy: Preliminary Communication', *Journal of Nervous and Mental Disease* 142, no. 2 (1966): 148.
Coleborne, Catharine, *Insanity, Identity and Empire: Immigrants and Institutional Confinement in Australia and New Zealand, 1873–1910*. Manchester University Press, 2015.
Coleborne, Catharine, *Madness in the Family: Insanity and Institutions in Australasian Colonial World, 1860–1914*. Routledge, 2009.
Collins, Brianne M., and Henderikus J. Stam, 'A Transnational Perspective on Psychosurgery: Beyond Portugal and the United States', *Journal of the History of the Neurosciences* 23, no. 4 (2014): 335–54.
Condrau, Flurin, 'The Patient's view Meets the Clinical Gaze', *Social History of Medicine* 20, no. 3 (2007): 225–40.

Cooter, Roger, ed., *In the Name of the Child: Health and Welfare, 1880–1940*. Routledge, 1992.
Cooter, Roger, 'Neural Veils and the Will to Historical Critique: Why Historians of Science Need to Take the Neuro-Turn Seriously', *Isis* 105 (2014): 145–54.
Corstens, Dirk, et al., 'Emerging Perspectives from the Hearing Voices Movement: Implications for Research and Practice', *Schizophrenia Bulletin* 40 (2014): S285–94.
Cosgrove, Lisa, et al., 'A Critical Review of the Lancet Commission on Global Mental Health and Sustainable Development: Time for a Paradigm Change', *Critical Public Health* 30 (2020): 624–31.
'The Country's Mental Health', *The Lancet* 230, no. 5957 (30 October 1937): 1036–37.
Crane, Johanna Tayloe, *Scrambling for Africa: AIDS, Expertise, and the Rise of American Global Health Science*. Cornell University Press, 2013.
Crozier, Ivan, and Emmanuel Delille, 'Introduction: Pow Meng Yap and the Culture-bound Syndromes', *History of Psychiatry* 29 (2018): 363–85.
Crutchfield, Parker, and Michael Redinger, 'The Conditions for Ethical Chemical Restraints', *AJOB Neuroscience* 15, no.1 (2024): 3–16.
Cueto, Marcos, Theodore M. Brown, and Elizabeth Fee, *The World History Organization: A History*. Cambridge University Press, 2019.
Cummins, Ian, *Mental Health Services and Community Care: A Critical History*. Bristol University Press, 2021.
Czech, Herwig, 'Hans Asperger, National Socialism, and "Race Hygiene" in Nazi-era Vienna', *Molecular Autism* 9, no. 29 (2018): 1–43.
Czech, Herwig, 'Response to "Non-complicit": Revisiting Hans Asperger's Career in Nazi-era Vienna', *JADD* 49 (2019): 3883–87.
Dadwal, Viva, Matthew Harris, and Shams Sye, eds., *Reverse Innovation in Global Health Systems: Learning from Low-income Countries*. BMC, online, www.biomedcentral.com/collections/reverseinnovations.
Dagfal, Alejandro A., 'Psychology and Psychoanalysis in Argentina: Politics, French Thought, and the University Connection, 1955–1976', *History of Psychology* 21 (2018): 254–72.
Dain, Norman, 'Critics and Dissenters: Reflections on "Anti-Psychiatry" in the United States', *Journal of the History of the Behavioural Sciences* 25, no. 1 (1989): 3–25.
Dalal, Farhad, *CBT: The Cognitive Behavioural Tsunami: Managerialism, Politics and the Corruptions of Science*. Routledge, 2018.
Daniels, D.N., et al., eds., *Violence and the Struggle for Existence*. Little, Brown and Company, 1970.
Danto, Elizabeth, *Freud's Free Clinics: Psychoanalysis and Social Justice, 1918–1938*. Columbia University Press, 2005.
D'Arrigo, T., 'On Its 50th Anniversary, BPA Looks Back on History and Ahead to Future', *Psychiatric News* 54, no. 10 (2019): 10.
Das, Anindya, and Mohan Rao, 'Universal Mental Health: Re-evaluating the Call for Global Mental Health', *Critical Public Health* 22, no. 4 (2012): 383–89.
David, D., et al., 'Why Cognitive Behavioral Therapy Is the Current Gold Standard of Psychotherapy', *Frontiers in Psychotherapy* 9, no. 4 (2018).
Davison, Kate, 'Cold War Pavlov: Homosexual Aversion Therapy in the 1960s', *History of the Human Sciences* 34, no. 1 (2021): 89–119.
Dax, E. Cunningham, *Asylum to Community: The Development of the Mental Hygiene Service in Victoria, Australia*. F.W. Cheshire, 1961.
Deaton, Angus, and Nancy Cartwright, 'Understanding and Misunderstanding Randomised Controlled Trials', *Social Science & Medicine* 210 (2018): 2–21.
'The Decade of the Brain', *Presidential Proclamation 6158*, 17 July 1990, www.loc.gov/loc/brain/proclaim.html.
Decker, Hannah, *The Making of DSM-III: A Diagnostic Manual's Conquest of American Psychiatry*. Oxford University Press, 2013.
Deleuze, Gilles, and Félix Guattari, *Anti-Oedipus: Capitalism and Schizophrenia*, trans. Robert Hurley, Mark Seem and Helen R. Lane. Penguin, 2009.

Deleuze, Gilles, and Félix Guattari, *A Thousand Plateaus*. Continuum, 2004.
Delille, Emmanuel, and Ivan Crozier, 'Historicizing Transcultural Psychiatry: People, Epistemic Objects, Networks, and Practices', *History of Psychiatry* 29 (2018): 257–62.
De Moore, Greg, and Ann Westmore, *Finding Sanity: John Cade, Lithium and the Taming of Bipolar Disorder*. Allen & Unwin, 2016.
Denholtz, Myron S., and Edward Mann, 'Automated Audiovisual Treatment of Phobias Administered by Nonprofessionals', *Journal of Behaviour Therapy and Experimental Psychiatry* 6 (1975): 111–15.
Denholtz, Myron S., and Edward Mann, 'Automated Treatment for Flight Phobia: A 3½-Year Follow-up', *American Journal of Psychiatry* 135, no. 11 (1978): 1340–43.
Derksen, Maarten, 'Turning Men into Machines? Scientific Management, Industrial Psychology, and the "Human Factor"', *Journal of the History of the Behavioral Sciences* 50, no. 2 (2014): 148–65.
Deutsch, Albert, *Shame of the States*. Harcourt, 1948.
Dibden, W.A., 'Prefrontal Leucotomy for Obsessional Neurosis: Report of a Case', *Medical Journal of Australia* (25 October 1947): 511–12.
Digby, Anne, *Madness, Morality and Medicine: A Study of the York Retreat*. Cambridge University Press, 1985.
Dooner, Caroline, *Tired as F*ck: Burnout at the Hands of Diet, Self-Help, and Hustle Culture*. Harper Wave, 2022.
Doroshow, Deborah Blythe, 'Performing a Cure for Schizophrenia: Insulin Coma Therapy on the Wards', *Journal of the History of Medicine and Allied Sciences* 62, no. 2 (2007): 213–43.
Dowbiggin, Ian, *Keeping American Sane: Psychiatry and Eugenics in the United States and Canada*. Cornell University Press, 2003.
Dowbiggin, Ian, *The Quest for Mental Health: A Tale of Science, Medicine, Scandal, Sorrow, and Mass Survival*. Cambridge University Press, 2011.
Doyle, D., 'A Load Off Whose Heart? Psychiatry and the Politics of Respectability and Race Representation in Harlem, 1943–45', *Journal of the History of Medicine and Allied Sciences* 75, no. 1 (2019): 54–82.
Draper, Brian, 'Older People in Hospitals for the Insane in New South Wales, Australia, 1849–1905', *History of Psychiatry* 32, no. 4 (2021): 436–48.
Drecker, Hannah, *The Making of DSM-III: A Diagnostic Manual's Conquest of American Psychiatry*. Oxford University Press, 2013.
Drescher, Jack, 'An Interview with Robert Spitzer', *Journal of Gay and Lesbian Psychotherapy* 7, no. 3 (2003): 97–111.
Drescher, Jack, 'Judd Marmor, Psychiatry and Homosexuality', *Journal of Gay & Lesbian Psychotherapy* 10, no. 2 (2006): 117–25.
Du Bois, W.E.B., *Black Reconstruction in America: An Essay Toward a History of the Part Which Black Folk Played in the Attempt to Reconstruct Democracy in America, 1860–1880*. Russell and Russell, [1935] 1966.
Dufaud, Grégory, and Lara Rzesnitzek, 'Soviet Psychiatry through the Prism of Circulation: The Case of Outpatient Psychiatry in the Interwar Period', *Kritika* 17, no. 4 (2016): 781–803.
Dumit, Joseph, 'Plastic Neuroscience: Studying What the Brain Cares About', *Frontiers in Human Neuroscience* 8 (2014): 176.
Dunk, James H., et al., 'Human Health on an Ailing Planet—Historical Perspectives on Our Future', *New England Journal of Medicine* 381 (2019): 778–82.
Dunlop, Robyn, and Hans Pols, 'Deinstitutionalisation and Mental Health Activism in Australia: Emerging Voices of Individuals with Lived Experience of Severe Mental Distress, 1975–1985', *History Australia* 19, no. 1 (2022): 92–114.
Durkheim, Émile, *Suicide: A Study in Sociology*, trans. John A. Spaulding and George Simpson. Free Press, 1951.

Durn, Tyler, 'Do No Harm in Due Process—A Historical Analysis of Social Determinates of Institutionalization in the USA', *History of Psychiatry* 32, no. 4 (2021): 478–87.

Eagar, Kathy, Anita Westera, and Conrad Kobel, 'Australian Residential Aged Care Is Understaffed', *Medical Journal of Australia* 212, no. 11 (2020): 507–08.e1.

Edele, M., and R. Gerwarth, 'The Limits of Demobilisation: Global Perspectives on the Aftermath of the Great War', *Journal of Contemporary History* 50, no. 1 (2015): 3–14.

Edington, Claire, *Beyond the Asylum: Mental Illness in French Colonial Vietnam*. Cornell University Press, 2019.

'Editorial: Mental Health of School Children', *Journal of the American Medical Association* XLVII, no. 1 (7 July 1906): 39–40

'Editorial Policy', *Human Relations* 1, no. 1 (1947): 1–2.

'Editorial: Pseudopatients', *British Medical Journal* (28 December 1974): 729–30.

'Editor's Notebook: Aggression and Violence', *American Journal of Psychiatry* 128, no. 4 (1971): 474.

Edwards, K.F., 'Four Cases of Prefrontal Leucotomy', *Medical Journal of Australia* (25 October 1947): 512–16.

Eghigian, Greg, 'Deinstitutionalizing the History of Contemporary Psychiatry', *History of Psychiatry* 22, no. 2 (2011): 201–14.

Ellis, Albert, 'Rational Psychotherapy', *Journal of General Psychology* 59 (1958): 35–49.

El Shakry, Omnia, *The Arabic Freud: Psychoanalysis and Islam in Modern Egypt*. Princeton University Press, 2017.

Elvevåg, Brita, et al., 'Quantifying Incoherence in Speech: An Automated Methodology and Novel Application to Schizophrenia', *Schizophrenia Research* 93 (2007): 304–16

Engstrom, Eric J., *Clinical Psychiatry in Imperial Germany: A History of Psychiatric Practice*. Cornell University Press, 2003.

Engstrom, Eric J., and Ivan Crozier, 'Race, Alcohol and General Paralysis: Emil Kraepelin's Comparative Psychiatry and His Trips to Java (1904) and North American (1925)', *History of Psychiatry* 29 (2018): 263–81.

Engstrom, Eric J., and Matthias M. Weber, 'Making Kraepelin History: A Great Instauration?', *History of Psychiatry* 18 (2007): 267–73.

Enns, Peter K., *Incarceration Nation: How the United States Became the Most Punitive Democracy in the World*. Cambridge University Press, 2016.

Erichsen, John, *On Railway and Other Injuries of the Nervous System*. Henry C. Lea, 1867.

Falk, Dean, 'More on Asperger's Career: A Reply to Czech', *JADD* 49 (2019): 3877–82.

Falk, Dean, 'Non-complicit: Revisiting Hans Asperger's Career in Nazi-era Vienna', *Journal of Autism and Developmental Disorders* 50 (2020): 2573–84.

Fanon, Frantz, 'Day Hospitalization in Psychiatry: Value and Limits' (1959) and (with Charles Geronimi), 'Day Hospitalization in Psychiatry: Value and Limits. Part Two: Doctrinal Considerations', in *Alienation and Freedom*, ed. Jean Khalfa and Robert J.C. Young, trans. Steven Corcoran. Bloomsbury Academic, 2018, pp. 473–509.

Fanon, Frantz, 'Letter to the Resident Minister', December 1956, in *Alienation and Freedom*, ed. Jean Khalfa and Robert J.C. Young, trans. Steven Corcoran. Bloomsbury Academic, 2018, p. 434.

Fanon, Frantz, *The Wretched of the Earth*, trans. Constance Farrington, Penguin, [1961] 1965.

Farahany, Nita A., *The Battle for Your Brain: Defending the Right to Think Freely in the Age of Neurotechnology*. St. Martin's Press, 2023.

Farley, John, *To Cast Out Disease: A History of the International Health Division of the Rockefeller Foundation (1913–1951)*. Oxford University Press, 2003.

Fassin, Didier, and Richard Rechtman, *The Empire of Trauma: An Inquiry into the Condition of Victimhood*, trans. Rachel Gomme. Princeton University Press, 2009.

Feldman, M.P., and M.J. MacCulloch, 'A Systematic Approach to the Treatment of Homosexuality by Conditioned Aversion: Preliminary Report', *American Journal of Psychiatry* 121, no. 2, (1964): 167–71.

Felitti, Vincent J., 'Origins of the ACE Study', *American Journal of Preventative Medicine* 56, no. 6 (2019): 787–89.
Fink, Max, 'Meduna and the Origins of Convulsive Therapy', *American Journal of Psychiatry* 141, no. 9 (1984): 1034–41.
Fishman, Jacob R., and John McCormack, '"Mental Health Without Walls": Community Mental Health in the Ghetto', *American Journal of Psychiatry* 126, no. 10 (1970): 1461–67.
Foot, John, *The Man Who Closed the Asylums: Franco Basaglia and the Revolution in Mental Health Care*. Verso, 2015.
'Foreword', *Mental Health* 1, no. 1 (January 1940): 1.
Forrester, John, *Dispatches from the Freud Wars: Psychoanalysis and Its Passions*. Harvard University Press, 1998.
Forrester, John, 'If p, Then Phat? Thinking in Cases', *History of the Human Sciences* 9, no. 3 (1996): 1–25.
Foucault, Michel, *The Birth of Biopolitics: Lectures at the Collège de France, 1978–1979*, trans. Graham Burchell. Palgrave, 2008.
Foucault, Michel, *Madness and Civilization: A History of Madness in the Age of Reason*. Pantheon, 1965.
Frances, Allen, *Saving Normal: An Insider's Revolt Against Out of Control Psychiatric Diagnosis, DSM-5, Big Pharma, and the Medicalization of Ordinary Life*. William Morrow, 2013.
Frank, I.M., and F.S. Hoedemaker, 'The Civilian Psychiatrist and the Draft', *American Journal of Psychiatry* 127, no. 4 (1970): 497–502.
Franklin, Isaac, et al., 'Theory-Driven Analysis of Natural Language Processing Measures of Thought Disorder Using Generative Language Modeling', *Biological Psychiatry: Cognitive Neuroscience and Neuroimaging* 8 (2023): 1013–23.
'Fraser House: Patients' Rules for Committees', in Neville T. Yeomans Papers, 1960–1971, State Library of New South Wales, MLMSS. 2416/2, Papers re Fraser House, 1960–1967.
'Fraser House Unit Rules—Visiting', in Neville T. Yeomans Papers, 1960–1971, State Library of New South Wales, MLMSS. 2416/2, Papers re Fraser House, 1960–1967.
Freedman, Estelle B., 'Uncontrollable Desires: The Response to the Sexual Psychopath', *Journal of American History* 74, no. 1 (1987): 83–106.
Freudenberger, Herbert J., 'Staff Burn-Out', *Journal of Social Issues* 30, no. 1 (1974): 159–65.
Freudenberger, Herbert J., 'The Staff Burn-out Syndrome in Alternative Institutions', *Psychotherapy: Theory, Research & Practice* 12, no. 1 (1975): 73–82.
Freudenberger, Herbert J., with Geraldine Richelson, *Burn-out: The High Cost of High Achievement*. Doubleday, 1980.
Freudenthal, Robert, and Joanna Moncrieff, '"A Landmark in Psychiatric Progress"? The Role of Evidence in the Rise and Fall of Insulin Coma Therapy', *History of Psychiatry* 33, no. 1 (2022): 65–78.
Friedlander, Henry, *Origins of the Nazi Genocide: From Euthanasia to the Final Solution*. University of North Carolina Press, 1995.
Friedli, Lynne, and Robert Stearn, 'Positive Affect as Coercive Strategy: Conditionality, Activation and the Role of Psychology in UK Government Workfare Programmes', *Medical Humanities* 41 (2015): 40–47.
Fromm, Erich, *Escape from Freedom*. Avon Books, 1965.
Fuchs, Thomas, 'Are Mental Illnesses Diseases of the Brain?', in *Critical Neuroscience: A Handbook of the Social and Cultural Contexts of Neuroscience*, ed. Suparna Choudhury and Jan Slaby. Wiley, 2011, pp. 331–44.
Fuechtner, Veronika, Douglas E. Haynes and Ryan M. Jones, eds., *A Global History of Sexual Science, 1880–1960*. University of California Press, 2018.
Fussinger, Catherine, '"Therapeutic Community", Psychiatry's Reformers and Antipsychiatrists: Reconsidering Changes in the Field of Psychiatry after World War II', *History of Psychiatry* 22, no. 2 (2011): 146–63.

Galea, Sandro, et al., 'Reparations as a Public Health Priority—A Strategy for Ending Black-White Health Disparities', *New England Journal of Medicine* 383 (2020): 2101–03.
Galmarini-Kabala, Maria Cristina, 'Psychiatry, Violence, and the Soviet Project of Transformation: A Micro-History of the Perm Psycho-Neurological School-Sanatorium', *Slavic Review* 77, no. 2 (2018): 307–32.
Gambino, Matthew, '"These Strangers within Our Gates": Race, Psychiatry and Mental Illness Among Black Americans at St Elizabeths Hospital in Washington, DC, 1900–40', *History of Psychiatry* 19, no. 4 (2008): 387–408.
Garcia, J., *Psychology Comes to Harlem: Rethinking the Race Question in Twentieth Century America*. Johns Hopkins University Press, 2012.
Gardiner, Judith Kegan, 'Can Ms Prozac Talk Back? Feminism, Drugs, and Social Constructionism', *Feminist Studies* 21, no. 3 (1995): 501–17.
Gaston, Shytierra, 'Historical Racist Violence and Intergenerational Harms: Accounts from Descendants of Lynching Victims', *Annals of the American Academy of Political and Social Science* 694 (2021): 78–91
Gauld, Christophe, 'From Psychiatric Kinds to Harmful Symptoms', *Synthese* 200 (2022): article 440.
Gault, W.B., 'Some Remarks on Slaughter', *American Journal of Psychiatry* 128, no. 4 (1971): 451.
Gay, Peter, *Freud: A Life for Our Time*. W.W. Norton, 2006.
Gee, Graham, et al., 'Aboriginal and Torres Strait Islander Social and Emotional Wellbeing', in *Working Together: Aboriginal and Torres Strait Islander Mental Health and Wellbeing Principles and Practice*, ed. Pat Dudgeon et al. 2nd ed. Commonwealth of Australia, 2014, pp. 55–58.
Geissmann, Pierre, and Claudine Geissmann, *A History of Child Psychoanalysis*. Routledge, 1998.
Gerard, Donald L., 'Chiarugi and Pinel Considered: Soul's Brain/Person's Mind', *Journal of the History of the Behavioural Sciences* 33, no. 4 (1997): 381–403.
Geroulanos, Stefanos, and Todd Meyers, *The Human Body in the Age of Catastrophe: Brittleness, Integration, Science, and the Great War*. University of Chicago Press, 2018.
Ghosh, Peter, *Max Weber and the Protestant Ethic: Twin Histories*. Oxford University Press, 2014.
Giami, Alain, and Sharman Levinson, eds., *Histories of Sexuality: Between Science and Politics*. Palgrave Macmillan, 2021.
Gigerenzer, Gerd, *Adaptive Thinking: Rationality in the Real World*. Oxford University Press, 2002.
Gill-Peterson, Jules, *Histories of the Transgender Child*. University of Minnesota Press, 2018.
Gitre, Edward J.K., 'Importing Freud: First-Wave Psychoanalysis, Interwar Social Sciences, and the Interdisciplinary Foundations of an American Social Theory', *Journal of the History of the Behavioural Sciences* 46, no. 3 (2010): 239–62.
Glickman, S.W., et al., 'Ethical and Scientific Implications of the Globalisation of Clinical Research', *New England Journal of Medicine* 360 (2009): 816–23.
Gnambs, Timo, and Kai Kaspar, 'Disclosure of Sensitive Behaviours Across Self-administered Survey Modes: A Meta-analysis', *Behaviour Research Methods* 47 (2015): 1237–59.
Goffman, Erving, *Asylums: Essays on the Social Situation of Mental Patients and Other Inmates*. Anchor Books, 1961.
Gold, Ronald, 'Stop It, You're Making Me Sick!', in R.J. Stoller et al., 'A Symposium: Should Homosexuality Be in the APA Nomenclature?', *American Journal of Psychiatry* 130, no. 11 (1973): 1212.
Goldman, Howard H., and Gerald N. Grob, 'Defining "Mental Illness" in Mental Health Policy', *Health Affairs* 25, no. 3 (2006): 737–49.
Gonaver, Wendy, *The Peculiar Institution and the Making of Modern Psychiatry, 1840–1880*. University of North Carolina Press, 2018.

Gone, Joseph P., 'The Impact of Historical Trauma on Health Outcomes for Indigenous Populations in the USA and Canada: A Systematic Review', *American Psychologist* 74, no. 1 (2019): 20–35.

Goodchild, Philip, *Deleuze and Guattari: An Introduction to the Politics of Desire*. Sage, 1996.

Green, Danielle, 'Mental Health is Political', *New York Times*, 20 September 2022.

Green, Huw, 'We Have Reached Peak "Mental Health"', *New York Times*, 23 September 2022.

Greenblatt, Milton, 'Towards a Definition of Psychopolitics', *Psychiatric Annals* 5, no. 10 (1975): 393–98.

Greenley, J.R., D.P. Gillespie and J.J. Lindenthal, 'A Race Riot's Effect on Psychological Symptoms', *Archives of General Psychiatry* 32, no. 9 (1975): 1189–95.

Grey, Flick, 'Benevolent Othering: Speaking Positively about Mental Health Service Users', *Philosophy, Psychiatry & Psychology* 23 (2016): 241–51.

Grier, W., and P. Cobbs, *Black Rage*. Basic Books, 1968.

Grinker, R.R., and J.P. Spiegel, *Men Under Stress*. Blakiston, 1945.

Grob, Gerald N., *From Asylum to Community: Mental Health Policy in Modern America*. Princeton University Press, 1991.

Grob, Gerald N., *Mental Illness and American Society, 1875–1940*. Princeton University Press, 1983.

Guenther, Katja, *Localization and Its Discontents: A Genealogy of Psychoanalysis and the Neuro Disciplines*. University of Chicago Press, 2015.

Guenther, Katja, '"Um, mm-h, Yeah": Carl Rogers, Phonographic Recordings, and the Making of Therapeutic Listening', *History of Psychology* 25, no. 3 (2022): 191–210.

Gunderson, J., ed., 'Letters to the Editor: Viet Nam: The Board of Trustees Steps Out of Bounds', *American Journal of Psychiatry* 130, no. 5 (1973): 610.

Guttmacher, Manfred S., 'The Homosexual in Court', *American Journal of Psychiatry* 112, no. 8 (1956): 591–98.

Hack, Karl, *The Malayan Emergency*. Cambridge University Press, 2021.

Hacking, Ian, 'Kinds of People: Moving Targets', *Proceedings of the British Academy* 151 (2007): 285–318.

Hackney, S., 'Southern Violence', *American Historical Review* 74, no. 3 (1969): 906–25.

Hale, Nathan G., *The Rise and Crisis of Psychoanalysis in the United States: Freud and the Americans, 1917–1985*. Oxford University Press, 1995.

Halliwell, Martin, 'Going Home: World War II and Demobilization', in *Therapeutic Revolutions: Medicine, Psychiatry, and American Culture, 1945–1970*. Rutgers University Press, 2013, pp. 17–47.

Halliwell, Martin, *Therapeutic Revolutions: Medicine, Psychiatry and American Culture, 1945–1970*. Rutgers University Press, 2013.

Han, Byung-Chul, *The Burnout Society*, trans. Erik Butler. Stanford University Press, 2015.

Han, Byung-Chul, *Psychopolitics: Neoliberalism and New Technologies of Power*, trans. Erik Butler. Verso, 2017.

Haney, Craig, 'The Psychological Effects of Solitary Confinement: A Systematic Critique', *Crime and Justice* 47 (2018): 365–416.

Hankerson, Sidney H., et al., 'The Intergenerational Impact of Structural Racism and Cumulative Trauma on Depression', *American Journal of Psychiatry* 179 (2022): 434–40.

Harrison, Tom, *Bion, Rickman, Foulkes and the Northfield Experiments: Advancing on a Different Front*. Jessica Kingsley Publishers, 2009.

Hauser, Tobias U., et al., 'The Promise of a Model-based Psychiatry: Building Computational Models of Mental Ill Health', *The Lancet: Digital Health* 11, no. 4 (October 2022), E816–E28.

Hayward, Rhodri, 'The Invention of the Psychosocial: An Introduction', *History of the Human Sciences* 25, no. 5 (2012): 3–12.

Healy, David, 'Antidepressants and Sexual Dysfunction: A History', *Journal of the Royal Society of Medicine* 113, no. 4 (2020): 133–35.

Healy, David, *Let Them Eat Prozac: The Unhealthy Relationship Between the Pharmaceutical Industry and Depression*. New York University Press, 2004.
Heaton, Matthew M., *Black Skin, White Coats: Nigerian Psychiatrists, Decolonization, and the Globalization of Psychiatry*. Ohio University Press, 2013.
Heberer, Patricia, 'The Nazi "Euthanasia" Program', in *Routledge History of the Holocaust*, ed. Jonathan C. Friedman. Routledge, 2011.
Henry, Brandy F., 'Disparities in Use of Disciplinary Solitary Confinement by Mental Health Diagnosis, Race, Sexual Orientation, and Sex: Results from a National Survey in the United States of America', *Criminal Behaviour & Mental Health* 32, no. 2 (2022): 114–23.
Herman, Judith Lewis, *Trauma and Recovery*. Basic Books, 2001.
Herzberg, David, *Happy Pills in America: From Miltown to Prozac*. Johns Hopkins University Press, 2009.
Herzog, Dagmar, *Cold War Freud: Psychoanalysis in an Age of Catastrophe*. Cambridge University Press, 2017.
Hess, Volker, and Benoît Majerus, 'Writing the History of Psychiatry in the 20th Century', *History of Psychiatry* 22, no. 2 (2011): 139–45.
Hide, Louise, *Gender and Class in English Asylums, 1890–1914*. Palgrave Macmillan, 2014.
Higgs, Rory Neirin, 'Reconceptualizing Psychosis: The Hearing Voices Movement and Social Approaches to Health', *Health and Human Rights Journal* 22, no. 1 (2020): 133–44.
Hill, J.M.M., and E.L. Trist, 'A Consideration of Industrial Accidents as Means of Withdrawal from the Work Situation', *Human Relations* 6, no. 4 (1953): 357–80.
Hillman, B.L., *Dressing for the Culture Wars: Style and the Politics of Self-Presentation in the 1960s and 1970s*. University of Nebraska Press, 2015.
Hinton, Elizabeth, *From the War on Poverty to the War on Crime*. Harvard University Press, 2017.
Hirshbein, Laura, and Sharmalie Sarvananda, 'History, Power, and Electricity: American Popular Magazine Accounts of Electroconvulsive Therapy, 1940–2005', *Journal of the History of the Behavioral Sciences* 44 (2008): 1–18.
Hoberman, J., *Black and Blue: The Origins and Consequences of Medical Racism*. University of California Press, 2012.
Hoffarth, Matthew J., 'The Making of Burnout: From Social Change to Self-awareness in the Postwar United States, 1970–82', *History of the Human Sciences* 30, no. 5 (2017): 35.
Hoffman, B., 'Health Care Reform and Social Movements in the United States', *American Journal of Public Health* 93, no. 1 (2003): 75–85.
Hollander, Nancy Caro, 'Psychoanalysts Bearing Witness: Trauma and Memory in Latin America', in *Psychoanalysis in the Barrios*, ed. Patricia Gherovici and Christopher Christian. Routledge, 2018, pp. 42–43.
Holm, Michael, *The Marshall Plan: A New Deal for Europe*. Routledge, 2017.
Honkasalo, Julian, 'When Boys Will *Not* Be Boys: American Eugenics and the Formation of Gender Nonconformity as Psychopathology', *NORMA* 11 (2016): 270–86.
Hooker, Evelyn, 'The Adjustment of the Male Overt Homosexual', *Journal of Projective Techniques* 21, no. 1 (1957): 18.
Horikawa, T., et al., 'Neural Decoding of Visual Imagery During Sleep', *Science* 340, no. 6132 (2013): 639–42.
Horkheimer, Max, and Theodor W. Adorno, *Dialectic of Enlightenment*. Allen Lane, 1973.
Horowitz, A.V., and G.N. Grob, 'The Troubled History of Psychiatry's Quest for Specificity', *Journal of Health Politics, Policy & Law* 41, no. 4 (2016): 521–39.
Horwitz, Allan V., *DSM: A History of Psychiatry's Bible*. Johns Hopkins University Press, 2021.
Howard, S., 'The Vietnam Warrior: His Experience, and Implications for Psychotherapy', *American Journal of Psychiatry* 30, no. 1 (1976): 121–35.
Hsueh-Hao Chiang, Howard, 'Effecting Science, Affecting Medicine: Homosexuality, the Kinsey Reports, and the Contested Boundaries of Psychopathology in the United States, 1948–1965', *Journal of the History of the Behavioural Science* 44, no. 4 (2008): 300–18.

Huertas, Rafael, 'Between Doctrine and Clinical Practice: Nosography and Semiology in the Work of Jean-Etienne-Dominique Esquirol (1772–1840)', *History of Psychiatry* 19, no. 2 (2008): 123–40.

Hughes, H.S., 'Emotional Disturbance and American Social Change, 1944–1969', *American Journal of Psychiatry* 126, no. 1 (1969): 21–28.

Hughes-Wilson, John, 'Pardons for All', *Royal United Services Institute for Defence Studies* 151, no. 5 (2006): 56–59.

Human Rights Watch, *'Fading Away': How Aged Care Facilities in Australia Chemically Restrain Older People with Dementia*. Human Rights Watch, 2019, www.hrw.org/report/2019/10/15/fading-away/how-aged-care-facilities-australia-chemically-restrain-older-people#_ftn58.

Hunt, R.A., *Pacification: The American Struggle for Vietnam's Hearts and Minds*. Westview Press, 1995.

Huys, Quentin J.M., et al., 'Advances in the Computational Understanding of Mental Illness', *Neuropsychopharmacology Reviews* 46 (2021): 3–19.

Ibrahim, Joseph E., 'COVID-19 and Residential Aged Care in Australia', *Australian Journal of Advanced Nursing* 37, no. 3 (2020).

Ilfeld, F.W., 'Overview of the Causes and Prevention of Violence', *Archives of General Psychiatry* 20, no. 6 (1969): 675–89.

Ingram, Richard A., 'A Genealogy of the Concept of "Mad Studies"', in *The Routledge International Handbook of Mad Studies*, ed. Peter Beresford and Jasna Russo. Routledge, 2021, pp. 93–97.

International Labour Organisation, 'ILO Declaration on Fundamental Principles and Rights at Work', *2022 Amendment*, www.ilo.org/wcmsp5/groups/public/—ed_norm/—declaration/documents/normativeinstrument/wcms_716594.pdf.

'The International Sanitary Conference, Paris, 1903', in *British Medical Journal* (12 December 1903): 1549–50.

Jacobsen, Michael Hviid, 'Introduction: Goffman Through the Looking Glass: From "Classical" to Contemporary Goffman', in *The Contemporary Goffman*, ed. Michael Hviid Jacobsen. Routledge, 2010.

Jahoda, Marie, *Current Concepts of Menta Health*. Basic Books, 1958.

Jain, Sanjeev, et al., 'Psychiatry in India: Historical Roots, Development as a Discipline and Contemporary Context', in *Mental Health in Asia and the Pacific: Historical and Cultural Perspectives*, ed. Harry Minas and Milton Lewis. Springer, 2017, pp. 39–55.

Jameson, Frederic, *Postmodernism, or The Cultural Logic of Late Capitalism*. Duke University Press, 1990.

Janssen, Diederik F., '*Melancholia Scytharum*: The Early Modern Psychiatry of Transgender Identification', *History of Psychiatry* 32 (2021): 270–88.

Jayawickrama, Janaka, and Jo Rose, 'Therapeutic Imperialism in Disaster and Conflict-affected Countries', in *The Routledge International Handbook of Critical Mental Health*, ed. Bruce Cohen. Routledge, 2018, pp. 213–23.

Jo, Eunkyung, et al., 'Exploring User Perspectives of and Ethical Experiences with Teletherapy Apps: Qualitative Analysis of User Reviews', *JMIR Mental Health* 10 (2023): e49684.

Johnson, David K., *The Lavender Scare: The Cold War Persecution of Gays and Lesbians in the Federal Government*. University of Chicago Press, 2004.

Johnson, Gordon, and Sam Gershon, 'Early North American Research on Lithium', *Australian and New Zealand Journal of Psychiatry* 33 (1999): S48–S53.

Johnson, W., and H. Corral, 'Statements about Viet Nam: APA's Role', *American Journal of Psychiatry* 130, no. 6 (1973): 721–22.

Jones, B.E., et al., 'Problems of Black Psychiatric Residents in White Training Institutes', *American Journal of Psychiatry* 127, no. 6 (1970): 798–803.

Jones, Edgar, and Shahina Rahman, 'The Maudsley Hospital and the Rockefeller Foundation: The Impact of Philanthropy on Research and Training', *Journal of the History of Medicine and Allied Science* 64, no. 3 (2008): 273–99.

Jones, Edgar, and Simon Wessely, *Shell Shock to PTSD: Military Psychiatry from 1900 to the Gulf War*. Psychology Press, 2005.

Jones, Maxwell, 'Rehabilitation of Forces Neurosis Patients to Civilian Life', *British Medical Journal* (6 April 1946): 533–35.

Jones, Tiffany Fawn, *Psychiatry, Mental Institutions, and the Mad in Apartheid South Africa*. Routledge, 2012.

Joseph, P.E., 'Introduction: Towards a Historiography of the Black Power Movement', in *The Black Power Movement: Rethinking the Civil Rights-Black Power Era*, ed. P.E. Joseph. Routledge, 2006, pp. 1–25.

Kapila, Shruti, 'The "Godless" Freud and His Indian Friends: An Indian Agenda for Psychoanalysis', in *Psychiatry and Empire*, ed. Sloan Mahone and Megan Vaughan. Palgrave MacMillan, 2007, pp. 124–52.

Kaufman, Bruce E., *Managing the Human Factor: The Early Years of Human Resource Management in American Industry*. Cornell University Press, 2019.

Keles, Betul, et al., 'A Systematic Review: The Influence of Social Media on Depression, Anxiety and Psychological Distress in Adolescents', *International Journal of Adolescence and Youth* 25, no. 1 (2020): 79–93.

Keller, Richard E., *Colonial Madness in French North Africa*. University of Chicago Press, 2007.

Keller, Richard E., 'Madness and Colonization: Psychiatry in the British and French Empires, 1800–1962', *Journal of Social History* 35, no. 2 (2001): 295–326.

Kelty-Stephenson, D.J., et al., 'In Search for an Alternative to the Computer Metaphor of the Mind and Brain', *arXiv*, arXiv:2206.04603.

Kendler, K.S., and J. Parnas, eds., *Philosophical Issues in Psychiatry: Explanation, Phenomenology, and Nosology*. Johns Hopkins University Press, 2008.

Kendler, K.S., P. Zachar, and C. Craver, 'What Kinds of Things Are Psychiatric Disorders?', *Psychological Medicine* 41 (2011): 1143–50.

Kennedy, Alexander, *Report to the Minister for Health on Mental Health and Mental Hygiene Services in the State of Victoria*. Government Printer, 1950.

Kerr, Matthew Newson, *Contagion, Isolation, and Biopolitics in Victorian London*. Palgrave, 2018.

Khanna, Ranjana, *Dark Continents: Psychoanalysis and Colonialism*. Duke University Press, 2003.

Kirmayer, Laurence J., 'Beyond the "New Cross-cultural Psychiatry": Cultural Biology, Discursive Psychology and the Ironies of Globalization', *Transcultural Psychiatry* 43 (2006): 126–44.

Klaf, Franklin S., and Charles A. Davis, 'Homosexuality and Paranoid Schizophrenia: A Survey of 150 Cases and Controls', *American Journal of Psychiatry* 116, no. 12 (1960): 1070–75.

Kleinman, Arthur M., 'Depression, Somatization and the "New Cross-Cultural Psychiatry"', *Social Science & Medicine* 11 (1977): 3–9.

Kleinman, Arthur M., 'Global Mental Health: A Failure of Humanity', *The Lancet* 374 (2009): 603–04.

Kohler-Hausmann, Julilly, *Getting Tough: Welfare and Imprisonment in 1970s America*. Princeton University Press, 2017.

Koppes, Bryan Laura, ed., *Historical Perspectives in Industrial and Organizational Psychology*. Routledge, 2020.

Korman, G.P., N. Viotti, and C.J. Garay, 'The Origins and Professionalisation of Cognitive Psychotherapy in Argentina', *History of Psychology* 18, no. 2 (2015): 205–14.

Kragh, Jesper Vaczy, *Lobotomy Nation: The History of Psychosurgery and Psychiatry in Denmark*. Palgrave, 2021.

Kramer, Barry Alan, 'Use of ECT in California, 1977–1983', *American Journal of Psychiatry* 142, no. 10 (1985): 1190–92.

Kramer, Peter D., *Listening to Prozac*. Fourth Estate, 1994.

Krantz, David S., et al., 'Post Traumatic Stress Disorder as a Systematic Disorder: Pathways to Cardiovascular Disease', *Health Psychology* 41, no. 10 (2022): 651–62.

Kremer, Malvina W., and Alfred H. Rifkin, 'The Early Development of Homosexuality: A Study of Adolescent Lesbians', *American Journal of Psychiatry* 126, no. 1 (1969): 91–96.

Kritsotaki, Despo, Vicky Long, and Mathew Smith, 'Introduction: Deinstitutionalisation and the Pathways of Post-War Psychiatry in the Western World', in *Deinstitutionalisation and After: Post-War Psychiatry in the Western World*, ed. Despo Kritsotaki, Vicky Long and Mathew Smith. Palgrave, 2016, pp. 22–29.

Laacke, Sebastian, et al., 'Artificial Intelligence, Social Media and Depression. A New Concept of Health-Related Digital Autonomy', *The American Journal of Bioethics* 21, no. 7 (2021): 4–20.

Laban, Guy, et al., 'Social Robots for Supporting Post-traumatic Stress Disorder Diagnosis and Treatment', *Frontiers in Psychiatry* 12 (2022): article 752874.

Ladd-Taylor, Molly, *Fixing the Poor: Eugenic Sterilization and Child Welfare in the Twentieth Century*. Johns Hopkins University Press, 2020.

Laffey, Paul, 'Antipsychiatry in Australia: Sources for a Social and Intellectual History', *Health and History* 5, no. 2 (2003): 26–28.

Lamb, H. Richard, and Linda E. Weinberger, 'Decarceration of U.S. Jails and Prisons: Where Will Persons with Serious Mental Illness Go?', *Journal of the American Academy of Psychiatry and the Law* 42, no. 4 (2014): 489–94.

Lamb, S.D., *Pathologist of the Mind: Adolf Meyer and the Origins of American Psychiatry*. Johns Hopkins University Press, 2014.

Lambe, Jennifer, 'Memory Politics: Psychiatric Critique, Cultural Protest, and *One Flew Over the Cuckoo's Nest*', *Literature and Medicine* 37, no. 2 (2019): 298–324.

LaMontagne, Anthony D., et al., 'Workplace Mental Health: Developing an Integrated Intervention Approach', *BMC Psychiatry* 14, no. 131 (2014).

Langner, H.P., 'The Making of a Murderer', *American Journal of Psychiatry* 127, no. 7 (1971): 950–53.

Lasch, Christopher, *The Culture of Narcissism: American Life in an Age of Diminishing Expectations*. Abacus, 1980.

Launer, John, 'Introduction', in *The Essential Writings of Sabina Spielrein*, trans. and ed. Ruth I. Cape and Raymond Burt. Routledge, 2018, pp. 1–13.

Leckie, Jaqueline, *Colonising Madness: Asylum and Community in Fiji*. University of Hawai'i Press, 2019.

Lee, Ellen E., et al., 'Artificial Intelligence for Mental Health Care: Clinical Applications, Barriers, Facilitators, and Artificial Wisdom', *Biological Psychiatry: Cognitive Neuroscience and Neuroimaging* 6, no. 9 (2021): 856–64.

Lejeune, Alban, et al., 'Artificial Intelligence and Suicide Prevention: A Systematic Review', *European Psychiatry* 17, no. 16 (2022): 5929.

Levant, Ronald F., 'Visit to the U.S. Joint Task Force Station at Guantanamo Bay: A First Person Account', *Military Psychology* 19 (2007): 2.

Levin, E.C., 'Evading the Realities of War?', *American Journal of Psychiatry* 124, no. 8 (1968): 1138.

Lewis, Milton, *Managing Madness: Psychiatry and Society in Australia 1788–1980*. AGPS Press, 1988.

Leys, Ruth, *The Ascent of Affect: Genealogy and Critique*. University of Chicago Press, 2017.

Leys, Ruth, *From Guilt to Shame: Auschwitz and After*. Princeton University Press, 2007.

Leys, Ruth, *Trauma: A Genealogy*. University of Chicago Press, 2000.

Lifton, R.J., *Death in Life: Survivors of Hiroshima*. University of North Carolina Press, 1991.

Lifton, R.J., *Home from the War: Vietnam Veterans—Neither Victims nor Executioners*. Simon and Schuster, 1973.

Lin, Grant L., et al., 'Resident and Fellow Unions: Collective Activism to Promote Well-being for Physicians in Training', *Journal of the American Medical Association* 328, no. 7 (2022): 619–20.

Lin, Yi-Tang, *Statistics and the Language of Global Health: Institutions and Experts in China, Taiwan, and the World, 1917–1960*. Cambridge University Press, 2022.

Linebaugh, Riley, 'Colonial Fragility: British Embarrassment and the So-called "Migrated Archives"', *Journal of Imperial and Commonwealth History* 50, no. 4 (2022): 729–56.

Linstrum, Erik, *Ruling Minds: Psychology in the British Empire*. Harvard University Press, 2016.

Littlewood, Roland, 'From Categories to Contexts: A Decade of the "New Cross-Cultural Psychiatry"', *British Journal of Psychiatry* 156 (1990): 308–09.

Long, Vicky, *Destigmatising Mental Illness? Professional Politics and Public Education in Britain, 1870–1970*. Manchester University Press, 2014.

Looi, Jeffery C.L., et al., 'Psychiatric Care Implications of the Aged Care Royal Commission: Putting the Cart Before the Horse', *ANZJP* 56, no. 1 (2022): 11–13.

Loughran, Tracy, *Shell-Shock and Medical Culture in First World War Britain*. Cambridge University Press, 2017.

Lowinger, P., 'Sex, Selma and Segregation: A Psychiatrist's View', *International Journal of Social Psychiatry* 14, no. 2 (1968): 119–24.

Lowinger, P., C. Darrow, and F. Huige, 'Case Study of the Detroit Uprising: The Troops and the Leaders', *Archives of General Psychiatry* 21, no. 1 (1969): 33–38.

Lucas, Gale M., et al., 'It's Only a Computer: Virtual Humans Increase Willingness to Disclose', *Computers in Human Behaviour* 37 (2014): 94–100.

Lucas, Gale M., et al., 'Reporting Mental Health Symptoms: Breaking Down Barriers to Care with Virtual Human Interviewers', *Frontiers in Robotics and AI* 51 (2017): 1–9.

Lukács, Georg, 'Reification and the Consciousness of the Proletariat', in *History and Class Consciousness: Studies in Marxist Dialectics*, trans. Rodney Livingstone. Merlin Press, 1971.

Lundin, Johan, et al., 'Using 360-degree Videos for Virtual Reality Exposure in CBT for Panic Disorder with Agoraphobia: A Feasibility Study', *Behavioural and Cognitive Psychotherapy* 50, no. 2 (2021): 158–70.

Macey, David, *Frantz Fanon: A Biography*. Picador, 2000.

MacKenzie, Charlotte, *Psychiatry for the Rich: A History of Ticehurst Private Asylum, 1792–1917*. Routledge, 1992.

Macklin, Ruth, 'Mental Health and Mental Illness: Some Problems of Definition and Conception Formation', *Philosophy of Science* (1972): 341–65.

MacLeish, Kenneth, 'On "Moral Injury": Psychic Fringes and War Violence', *History of the Human Sciences* 31, no. 2 (2018): 128–46.

Madigan, Daniel J., and Lisa E. Kim, 'Towards an Understanding of Teacher Attrition: A Meta-analysis of Burnout, Job Satisfaction, and Teachers' Intentions to Quit', *Teaching and Teacher Education* 104 (2021): 103425.

Mahone, Sloan, and Megan Vaughan, 'Introduction', *Psychiatry and Empire*, ed. Sloan Mahone and Megan Vaughan. Palgrave MacMillan, 2007, pp. 1–16.

Mahoney, Gerald M., 'Unidimensional Scales for the Measurement of Morale in an Industrial Situation', *Human Relations* 9, no. 1 (1956): 3–26.

Maier, T., 'The Army Psychiatrist—An Adjunct to the System of Social Control', *American Journal of Psychiatry* 126, no. 7 (1970): 1039.

Makari, George, *Revolution in Mind: The Creation of Psychoanalysis*. Duckworth Overlook, 2010.

Malitz, Sidney, et al., 'A Two-Year Evaluation of Chlorpromazine in Clinical Research and Practice', *American Journal of Psychiatry* 113 (1956): 544–45.

Marcuse, Herbert, *One-dimensional Man: Studies in the Ideology of Advanced Industrial Society*. Routledge, 2002.

Marek, Scott, et al., 'Reproducible Brain-wide Association Studies Require Thousands of Individuals', *Nature* 603 (2022): 654–60.

Mark, Sprevak, and Matteo Colombo, eds., *The Routledge Handbook of the Computational Mind*. Routledge, 2019.

Marmor, Judd, 'Homosexuality and Cultural Value Systems', in R.J. Stoller et al., 'A Symposium: Should Homosexuality Be in the APA Nomenclature?', *American Journal of Psychiatry* 130, no. 11 (1973): 1209.

Martin, Jay, *The Dialectical Imagination: A History of the Frankfurt School and the Institute for Social Research, 1923–1950*. University of California Press, 1973.

Martín-Baró, Ignacio, *Writings for a Liberation Psychology*, ed. Adrianne Aron and Shawn Corne. Harvard University Press, 1996.

Marx, Karl, *Capital: A Critique of Political Economy, Volume One*, trans. Ben Fowkes. Penguin, 1976.

Maslach, Christina, *Burnout, the Cost of Caring*. Prentice-Hall Press, 1986.

Matassi, Giorgio, et al., 'Editorial: Current Thoughts on the Brain—Computer Analogy—All Metaphors Are Wrong, But Some Are Useful', *Frontiers in Ecology and Evolution* 11 (2023): 1–3.

Matlin, D., 'Who Speaks for Harlem? Kenneth B. Clark, Albert Murray, and the Controversies of Black Urban Life', *Journal of American Studies* 46, no. 4 (2012): 875–94.

Max-Planck-Gesellschaft, 'Epigenetics Between the Generations: We Inherit More than Just Genes', *ScienceDaily*, www.sciencedaily.com/releases/2017/07/170717100548.htm.

McCarthy, John F., et al., 'Evaluation of the Recovery Engagement and Coordination for Health—Veterans Enhanced Treatment Suicide Risk Modelling Clinical Program in the Veterans Health Administration', *Journal of the American Medical Association* 4, no. 10 (2021): 1–11.

McCarthy, John F., et al., 'Predictive Modeling and Concentration of the Risk of Suicide: Implications for Preventive Interventions in the US Department of Veterans Affairs', *American Journal of Public Health* 105, no. 9 (2015): 1935–42.

McConkey, Matthew, 'Human Animals: Moral Treatment and the Non-Human at York Retreat', *Literature and Medicine* 40, no. 2 (2022): 269–94.

Mccrae, Niall, '"A Violent Thunderstorm": Cardiazol Treatment in British Mental Hospitals', *History of Psychiatry* 17 (2006): 67–90.

McFarlane, Alexander C., 'Post-Traumatic Stress Disorder Is a Systemic Illness, Not a Mental Disorder: Is Cartesian Dualism Dead?', *Medical Journal of Australia* 206, no. 6 (2017): 248–49.

McGeachan, Cheryl, '"The World Is Full of Big Bad Wolves": Investigating the Experimental Therapeutic Spaces of R.D. Laing and Aaron Esterson', *History of Psychiatry* 25, no. 3 (2014): 283–98.

McGoey, Linsey, 'Profitable Failure: Anti-depressant Drugs and the Triumph of Flawed Experiments', *History of the Human Sciences* 23 (2010): 58–78.

McGrath, Larry S., 'Historiography, Affect, and the Neurosciences', *History of Psychology* 20 (2017): 129–47.

McNeil, J.R., 'Peak Document and the Future of History', *American Historical Review* 125 (2020): 1–18.

Mendes, Gabriel N., *Under the Strain of Color: Harlem's Lafargue Clinic and the Promise of an Antiracist Psychiatry*. Cornell University Press, 2015.

Menninger, K., 'New Violence and the New Psychiatry', *Bulletin of the Menninger Clinic* 32, no. 6 (1968): 341–54.

'Mental Health and Disease', *British Medical Journal* 2, no. 3541 (17 November 1928): 903–04.

'Mental Health and Social Problems', *BMJ* 2, no. 3592 (9 November 1929): 863–64.

'Mental Health as a National Problem', *Journal of the American Medical Association* 96, no. 13 (28 March 1931): 994–96.

'The Mental Health of the School Child', *Journal of the American Medical Association* LXIII, no. 14 (1914): 1225.

'Mental Health in 1929: Report of the Board of Control', *The Lancet* 216, no. 5586 (20 September 1930).

'Mental Health: Its Principles and Practice, with Emphasis on the Treatment of Mental Deviations', *Journal of the American Medical Association* 105, no. 7 (1935): 536.

'Mental Health of the Child', *Journal of the American Medical Association* 91, no. 5 (4 August 1928): 345.

'Mental Treatment Act, 1930: Prepared by the Board of Control', *British Medical Journal* (10 September 1930): 139–41.

Merksey, Harold, and Bronislava Shafran, 'Political Hazards in the Diagnosis of "Sluggish Schizophrenia"', *British Journal of Psychiatry* 148 (1986): 247–56.

Metzger, Marie-Hélène, et al., 'Use of Emergency Department Electronic Medical Records for Automated Epidemiological Surveillance of Suicide Attempts: A French Pilot Study', *International Journal of Methods in Psychiatric Research* 26, no. 2 (2017): e1522.

Metzger, Sean L., et al., 'A High-performance Neuroprosthesis for Speech Decoding and Avatar Control', *Nature* 620 (2023): 1037–46.

Metzl, Jonathan Michel, *Prozac on the Couch: Prescribing Gender in the Era of Wonder Drugs*. Duke University Press, 2003.

Metzner, Jeffrey L., and Jamie Fellner, 'Solitary Confinement and Mental Illness in U.S. Prisons: A Challenge for Medical Ethics', *Journal of the American Academy of Psychiatry and the Law* 38, no. 1 (March 2010): 104–08.

Meyer, Adolf, 'The Fourteenth Maudsley Lecture: British Influences in Psychiatry and Mental Hygiene', *Journal of Mental Science* 79 (1933): 458.

Meyer, Manuella, 'Sanity in the South Atlantic: The Mythos of Philippe Pinel and the Asylum Movement in Nineteenth-century Rio de Janeiro', *Atlantic Studies* 7 (2010): 473–92.

Micale, Mark, *Hysterical Men: The Hidden History of Male Nervous Illness*. Harvard University Press, 2008.

Micale, Mark, ed., *Traumatic Pasts in Asia: History, Psychiatry, and Trauma from the 1930s to the Present*. Berghahn Books, 2021.

Miller, P.R., 'Social Activists and Social Change: The Chicago Demonstrators', *American Journal of Psychiatry* 126, no. 12 (1970): 1752–59.

Mills, China, *Decolonizing Global Mental Health: The Psychiatrization of the Majority World*. Routledge, 2014.

Milne-Smith, Amy, 'Gender and Madness in Nineteenth-century Britain', *History Compass* 20, no. 11 (2022): e12754

Moncrieff, Joanna, et al., 'The Serotonin Hypothesis of Depression: Both Long Discarded and Still Supported', *Molecular Biology* 28, No. 8 (2023): 3160–63.

Moncrieff, Joanna, et al., 'The Serotonin Theory of Depression: A Systematic Umbrella Review of the Evidence', *Molecular Psychiatry* 28, no. 8 (2022): 3243–56.

Montague, P. Read, et al., 'Computational Psychiatry', *Trends in Cognitive Sciences* 16 (2012): [x]

Moon, Graham, Robin Kearns, and Alun Joseph, *Afterlives of the Psychiatric Asylum: Recycling Concepts, Sites and Memories*. Routledge, 2015.

Moore, Robert A., and Melvin L. Selzer, 'Male Homosexuality, Paranoia, and the Schizophrenias', *American Journal of Psychiatry* 119, no. 8 (1963): 743–47.

Mora, George, 'Vincenzo Chiarugi (1759–1820) and His Psychiatric Reform in Florence in the Late 18th Century', *Journal of the History of Medicine and Allied Sciences* 14, no. 10 (1959): 424–33.

Moran, James, *Committed to the State Asylum: Insanity and Society in Nineteenth-Century Quebec and Ontario*. McGill-Queen's University Press, 2000.

Morris, Nathaniel P., and Jacob M. Izenberg, 'Nowhere Else to Go—Solitary Confinement as Mental Health Care', *Journal of the American Medical Association* 330, no. 1 (2023): 17–18.

Moskowitz, J.A., 'On Drafting the Psychiatric "Draft" Letter', *American Journal of Psychiatry* 128, no. 1 (1971): 69–72.

Muheim, Flavio, 'Burnout: History of a Phenomenon', in *Burnout for Experts: Prevention in the Context of Living and Working*, ed. S. Bährer-Kohler. Springer, 2013, pp. 37–46.

Murphy, H.B.M., 'A Cross-Cultural Survey of Schizophrenic Symptomatology', *International Journal of Social Psychiatry* 9, no. 4 (1963): 237–49.

Murphy, H.B.M., et al., 'Crosscultural Inquiry into the Symptomatology of Depression: A Preliminary Report', *Transcultural Psychiatric Research Review and Newsletter* 1, no. 2 (1964): 5–18.

Musiat, P., and N. Tarrier, 'Collateral Outcomes in e-Mental Health: A Systematic Review of the Evidence for Added Benefits of Computerised Cognitive Behaviour Therapy Interventions for Mental Health', *Psychological Medicine* 44, no. 15 (2014): 3137–50.

Myers, E., 'Beyond the Psychological Wage: Du Bois on White Dominion', *Political Theory* 47, no. 1 (2019): 6–31.

Nadon, Lindsey, et al., 'Should Burnout Be Conceptualized as a Mental Disorder?', *Behavioral Sciences* 12, no. 82 (2022): 1.

Nagoski, Emily, and Amelia Nagoski, *Burnout: The Secret to Unlocking the Stress Cycle*. Ballantine Books, 2020.

Natale, Simone, 'The ELIZA Effect: Joseph Weizenbaum and the Emergence of Chatbots', in *Deceitful Media: Artificial Intelligence and Social Life after the Turing Test*. Oxford Academic, 2021, pp. 60–65.

'The National Mental Health and the War', *Journal of Mental Science* 48, no. 200 (January 1902): 73–74.

Nelson, A., *Body and Soul: The Black Panther Party and the Fight Against Medical Discrimination*. University of Minnesota Press, 2011.

Neuendorf, Mark, *Emotions and the Making of Psychiatric Reform in Britain, c.1770–1820*. Palgrave, 2021.

Nour, Matthew M., et al., 'Functional Neuroimaging in Psychiatry and the Case for Failing Better', *Neuron* 110 (2022): 2531.

'Official Actions: Highlights of the 124th Annual Meeting', *American Journal of Psychiatry* 128, no. 1 (1971): 137–40.

'Official Actions: Report of the Trustees' Policy Meeting March 1971', *American Journal of Psychiatry* 128, no. 3 (1971): 386.

Ögren, Kenneth, and Mikael Sandlun, 'Psychosurgery in Sweden 1944–1964', *Journal of the History of the Neurosciences* 14 (2005): 353–67.

Oliver, K., *The My Lai Massacre in American History and Memory*. Manchester University Press, 2006.

Ondaatje, M.L., *Black Conservative Intellectuals in Modern America*. University of Pennsylvania Press, 2010.

Oppenheim, Janet, *'Shattered Nerves': Doctors, Patients, and Depression in Victorian England*. Oxford University Press, 1991.

Owen, Alan, and Robin Winkler, 'General Practitioners and Psychosocial Problems: An Evaluation Using Pseudopatients', *Medical Journal of Australia* 2 (14 September 1974): 393–98.

Packard, Randall M., *A History of Global Health: Interventions into the Lives of Other People*. Johns Hopkins University Press, 2016.

Pagés, Max, 'The Sociotherapy of the Enterprise: The Condition of Psycho-social Change in Industrial Concerns and the Role of the Social Psychologist as an Agent of Social Change', *Human Relations* 12, no. 4 (1959): 31–34.

Palaniyappan, Lena, 'More Than a Biomarker: Could Language Be a Biosocial Marker of Psychosis?', *NPJ Schizophrenia* 42 (2021): 1–5.

Panch, Trishan, et al., 'Artificial Intelligence and Algorithmic Bias: Implications for Health Systems', *Journal of Global Health* 9, no. 2 (2019): 010318.

Parker, Gordon, Gabriela Tavella, and Kerrie Eyers, *Burnout: A Guide to Identifying Burnout and Pathways to Recovery*. Allen & Unwin, 2021.

Parsons, Anne, *From Asylum to Prison: Deinstitutionalisation and the Rise of Mass Incarceration after 1945*. University of North Carolina Press, 2018.

Paul, Diane B., 'Reflections on the Historiography of American Eugenics: Trends, Fractures, Tensions', *Journal of the History of Biology* 49 (2016): 641–58.

Penny, David, 'Epigenetics, Darwin, and Lamarck', *Genome Biology and Evolution* 7 (2015): 1758–60.

Penrose, L.S., 'Mental Disease and Crime: Outline of a Comparative Study of European Statistics', *British Journal of Medical Psychology* 18, no. 1 (1939): 1–15.

Petersen, Anne Helen, *Can't Even: How Millennials Became the Burnout Generation*. Random House, 2022.

Petocz, Agnes, 'The Scientific Status of Psychoanalysis Revisited', in *Philosophy, Science, and Psychoanalysis: A Critical Meeting*, ed. Simon Boag, Linda A.W. Brakel and Velsa Talvitie. Routledge, 2015, pp. 145–92.

Petryna, Adriana, *When Experiments Travel: Clinical Trials and the Global Search for Human Subjects*. Princeton University Press, 2009.

Philips, I., et al., 'The Psychiatrist, the APA, and Social Issues: A Symposium', *American Journal of Psychiatry* 128, no. 6 (1971): 677.

Phoenix, D.L., *The Anger Gap: How Race Shapes Emotion in Politics*. Cambridge University Press, 2019.

Pincock, Stephen, 'Tsung-yi Lin: Obituary', *The Lancet* 377, no. 9763 (2011): 376.

Plant, Rebecca Jo, *Mom: The Transformation of Motherhood in Modern America*. University of Chicago Press, 2010.

Plotkin, Mariano Ben, 'Freud and the Latin Americans: A Forgotten Relationship', in *Psychoanalysis in the Barrios: Race, Class, and the Unconscious*, ed. Patricia Gherovici and Christopher Christian. Routledge, 2018, pp. 21–37.

Plotkin, Mariano Ben, 'Freudian Slips: On the Complicated—and Lingering—Legacy of Psychoanalysis in Argentina', *World Policy Journal* 35, no. 1 (2018): 16–22.

Pols, Hans, *Nurturing Indonesia: Medicine and Decolonisation in the Dutch East Indies*. Cambridge University Press, 2018.

Ponturo, Ali, and Meegan Kilcullen, 'A Systematic Review of Evidence-based Psychological Interventions and Aboriginal and Torres Strait Islander People', *Clinical Psychologist* 25, no. 2 (2021): 198–211.

Porter, Dorothy, *Health, Civilization and the State: A History of Public Health from Ancient to Modern Times*. Routledge, 1999.

Porter, Roy, 'The Patient's View: Doing Medical History from Below', *Theory and Society* 14, no. 2 (1985): 175–98.

Porter, Roy, and David Wright, eds., *The Confinement of the Insane. International Perspectives, 1800–1965*. Cambridge University Press, 2003.

Porter, Theodore M., *Genetics in the Madhouse: The Unknown History of Human Heredity*. Princeton University Press, 2018.

Porter, Theodore M., *Trust in Numbers: The Pursuit of Objectivity in Science and Public Life*. Princeton University Press, 2020.

'Position Statement on Alternatives to Violence', *American Journal of Psychiatry* 126, no. 10 (1970): 1550.

'Position Statement on Homosexuality and Civil Rights', *American Journal of Psychiatry* 131, no. 4 (1974): 497.

'Position Statement on the Training of Minority Psychiatrists', *American Journal of Psychiatry* 128, no. 2 (1971): 257.

Poskett, James, *Materials of the Mind: Phrenology, Race, and the Global History of Science, 1815–1920*. University of Chicago Press, 2019.

Powell, Enoch, 'Address to the National Association of Mental Health Annual Conference, 9 March 1961', www.nuffieldtrust.org.uk/sites/default/files/2019-11/nhs-history-book/58-67/powell-s-water-tower-speech.html.

Pressman, Jack D., *Last Resort: Psychosurgery and the Limits of Medicine*. Cambridge University Press, 1998.

Pringle, Yolana, *Psychiatry and Decolonisation in Uganda*. Palgrave, 2019.
Prins, Seth J., 'Does Transinstitutionalisation Explain the Overrepresentation of People with Serious Mental Illnesses in the Criminal Justice System?', *Community Mental Health Journal* 47, no. 6 (2011): 716–22.
Prins, Seth J., 'Prevalence of Mental Illnesses in U.S. State Prisons: A Systematic Review', *Psychiatric Services* 65, no. 7 (2014): 866.
Proctor, Hannah, *Burnout: The Emotional Experience of Political Defeat*. Verso, 2024.
Proctor, Hannah, '"A Country Beyond the Pleasure Principle": Alexander Luria, Death Drive and Dialectic in Soviet Russia, 1917–1930', *Psychoanalysis & History* 18, no. 2 (2016): 155–82.
'Psychiatrist Concedes Sirhan Has "Substantial Mental Illness"', *The New York Times*, 4 April 1969: 31.
Ptashne, Mark, 'Epigenetics: Core Misconcept', *PNAS* 110 (2013): 7101–03.
Pykett, Jessica, and Byrony Enright, 'Geographies of Brain Culture: Optimism and Optimisation in Workplace Training Programmes', *Cultural Geographies* 23, no. 1 (2016): 51–68.
Rachman, S., 'Sexual Disorders and Behaviour Therapy', *American Journal of Psychiatry* 118, no. 3 (1961): 235–40.
Rainey, Stephen, et al., 'Brain Recording, Mind-reading, and Neurotechnology: Ethical Issues from Consumer Devices to Brain-based Speech Decoding', *Science and Engineering Ethics* 26, no. 4 (2020): 2295–311.
Raitt, Suzanne, 'Early British Psychoanalysis and the Medico-Psychological Clinic', *History Workshop Journal* 58 (2004): 63–85.
Ramezani, Niloofar, 'The Relationship Between Community Public Health, Behavioral Health Service Accessibility, and Mass Incarceration', *BMC Health Services Research* 22 (2022): article 966.
Raz, Mical, *The Lobotomy Letters: The Making of American Psychosurgery*. University of Rochester Press, 2013.
Raz, Mical, *What's Wrong with the Poor? Psychiatry, Race, and the War on Poverty*. University of North Carolina Press, 2013.
Read, Jason, 'A Genealogy of Homo-Economicus: Neoliberalism and the Production of Subjectivity', *Foucault Studies* 6 (2009): 25–36.
Reaume, Geoffrey, 'How Is Mad Studies Different from Anti-Psychiatry and Critical Psychiatry?', in *The Routledge International Handbook of Mad Studies*, ed. Peter Beresford and Jasna Russo. Routledge, 2021, pp. 98–107.
Reddy, William M., 'Neuroscience and the Fallacies of Functionalism', *History & Theory* 49 (2010): 412–25.
Reddy, William M., 'The Unavoidable Intentionality of Affect: The History of Emotions and the Neurosciences of the Present Day', *Emotion Review* 12 (2020): 168–78.
Reger, Mark A., et al., 'Patient Feedback on the Use of Predictive Analytics for Suicide Prevention', *Psychiatric Services* 72, no. 2 (2021): 129–35.
Reich, Rebecca, *State of Madness: Psychiatry, Literature, and Dissent after Stalin*. Northern Illinois University Press, 2018.
Reiff, Collin M., et al., 'Psychedelic-Assisted Psychotherapy', *American Journal of Psychiatry* 177 (2020): 391–420.
Reiter, Keramet, 'Experimentation on Prisoners: Persistent Dilemmas in Rights and Regulations', *California Law Review* 97, no. 2 (2009): 501–66.
Reiter, Keramet, et al., 'Psychological Distress in Solitary Confinement: Symptoms, Severity, and Prevalence in the United States, 2017–2018', *American Journal of Public Health* 110, Suppl 1 (2020): S56–S62.
'Report to the Special Committee of the Board of Directors of the American Psychological Association: Independent Review Relating to APA Ethics Guidelines, National Security Interrogations, and Torture', 2015, 9, https://www.apa.org/independent-review.
Richert, Lucas, *Break on Through: Radical Psychiatry and the American Counterculture*. The MIT Press, 2019.

Richert, Lucas, '"Therapy Means Political Change, Not Peanut Butter": American Radical Psychiatry, 1968–1975', *Social History of Medicine* 27, no. 1 (2014): 112–13.
Rieff, Philip, *The Triumph of the Therapeutic: Uses of Faith After Freud*. Penguin, 1973.
Ringer, Fritz, *Max Weber: An Intellectual Biography*. University of Chicago Press, 2004.
Robcis, Camille, *Disalienation: Politics, Philosophy, and Radical Psychiatry in Postwar France*. University of Chicago Press, 2021.
Roberts, Lewis R., et al., 'Unmet Needs in Oncology Clinical Research and Treatment in Africa: Focus on Ghana', *The Oncologist* 27, no. 9 (2022): 760–67.
Roberts-Pedersen, Elizabeth, 'POWs into Citizens: Repatriation, Gender, and the Civilian Resettlement Units in Great Britain', in *Gender and Trauma Since 1900*, ed. Paula A. Michaels and Christina Twomey. Bloomsbury, 2021, pp. 101–21.
Roberts-Pedersen, Elizabeth, 'Towards a (Bio)cultural History of the Brain?', *History Australia* 19 (2022): 151–60.
Robson, Belinda, '"He Made Us Feel Special": Eric Cunningham Dax, Edith Pardy and the Reform of Mental Health Services in Victoria, 1950s and 1960s', *Australian Historical Studies* 122 (2003): 270–89.
Rondinone, Troy, *Nightmare Factories: The Asylum in the American Imagination*. Johns Hopkins University Press, 2019.
Rose, Diana, 'Critical Qualitative Research on "Madness": Knowledge Making and Activism Among Those Designated "Mad"', *Wellcome Open Research* 6 (2021): 1–22.
Rose, Diana, 'Service User/Survivor-led Research in Mental Health: Epistemological Possibilities', *Disability & Society* 32 (2017): 773–89.
Rose, Diana, and Jayasree Kalathil, 'Power, Privilege and Knowledge: The Untenable Promise of Co-production in Mental "Health"', *Frontiers in Sociology* 4 (2019): 1–11.
Rose, Diana, and Nikolas Rose, 'Is "Another" Psychiatry Possible?', *Psychological Medicine* 53, no. 1 (2023): 49.
Rose, Jacqueline, 'Freud in the "Tropics"', *History Workshop Journal* 47 (1999): 49–67.
Rose, Nikolas, and Joelle M. Abi-Rached, *Neuro: The New Brain Sciences and the Management of the Mind*. Princeton University Press, 2013.
Rosen, Albert, 'Detection of Suicidal Patients: An Example of Some Limitations in the Prediction of Infrequent Events', *Journal of Consulting Psychology* 18, no. 6 (1954): 397–403.
Rosen, George, *A History of Public Health*. MD Publications, 1958
Rosen, Gerald M., 'Revisiting the Origins of EMDR', *Journal of Contemporary Psychotherapy* 53 (2023): 289–96.
Rosenhan, D.L., 'On Being Sane in Insane Places', *Science* 179 (1973): 250.
Rosner, Rachel I., 'Manualizing Psychotherapy: Aaron T. Beck and the Origins of *Cognitive Theory of Depression*', *European Journal of Psychotherapy and Counselling* 20 (2018): 25–47.
Rosner, Rachel I., 'The "Splendid Isolation" of Aaron T. Beck', *Isis* 105, no. 4 (2014): 734–58.
Ross, Dorothy, 'Freud and the Vicissitudes of Modernism in the United States, 1940–1980', in *After Freud Left: A Century of Psychoanalysis in America*, ed. John Burnham. Chicago University Press, 2012, pp. 185–88.
Rotenstein, Lisa S., et al., 'Prevalence of Burnout Among Physicians: A Systematic Review', *Journal of the American Medical Association* 320, no. 11 (2018): 1131–50.
Royal Commission into Aged Care Quality and Safety, *Final Report—List of Recommendations*, March 2021, 252, https://www.royalcommission.gov.au/aged-care/final-report.
Royal Commission into Defence and Veteran Suicide, *Interim Report*, 11 August 2022, https://defenceveteransuicide.royalcommission.gov.au/publications/royal-commission-defence-and-veteran-suicide-interim-report.
Ryalls, Emily D., and Sharon R. Mazzarella, '"Famous, Beloved, Reviled, Respected, Feared, Celebrated": Media Construction of Greta Thunberg', *Communication, Culture and Critique* 14 (2021): 438–53.

Sadowsky, Jonathan, 'Before and After Prozac: Psychiatry as Medicine, and the Historiography of Depression', *Culture, Medicine, and Psychiatry* 45 (2021): 479–502.
Sadowsky, Jonathan, *Electroconvulsive Therapy in America: The Anatomy of a Medical Controversy*. Routledge, 2016.
Sadowsky, Jonathan, *The Empire of Depression: A New History*. Polity, 2021.
'Safeguarding Mental Health', *Journal of the American Medical Association* 109, no. 17 (23 October 1937): 1391.
Saghir, Marcel T., et al., 'Homosexuality: III. Psychiatric Disorders and Disability in the Male Homosexual', *American Journal of Psychiatry* 126, no. 8 (1970): 1079–86.
Saghir, Marcel T., et al., 'Homosexuality. IV. Psychiatric Disorders and Disability in the Female Homosexual', *American Journal of Psychiatry* 127, no. 2 (1970): 147–54.
Sajno, Elena, et al., 'Machine Learning in Biosignals Processing for Mental Health: A Narrative Review', *Frontiers in Psychology* 13 (2022): 1–24.
Sanderson, Michael, et al., 'Predicting Death by Suicide Following an Emergency Department Visit for Parasuicide with Administrative Health Care System Data and Machine Learning', *eClinicalMedicine* 20 (2020): 1–9.
Sareyan, Alex, *The Turning Point: How Men of Conscience Brought About Major Change in the Care of America's Mentally Ill*. American Psychiatric Press, 1994.
Savelli, Mat, and Sarah Marks, 'Introduction', in *Psychiatry in Communist Europe*, ed. Mat Savelli and Sarah Marks. Palgrave, 2015, pp. 7–9.
Schacht, Anastassiya, 'Power in Psychiatry: Soviet Peer and Lay Hierarchies in the Context of Political Abuse of Psychiatry', *History of Psychiatry* 33, no. 1 (2022): 21–33.
Schatzberg, Alan F., 'Some Comments on Psychedelic Research', *American Journal of Psychiatry* 177 (2020): 368–69.
Schaufeli, Wilmar B., 'Burnout: A Short Socio-Cultural History', in *Burnout, Fatigue, Exhaustion*, ed. S. Neckel et al. Palgrave, 2017, pp. 105–27.
Schoonover, Carl E., *Portraits of the Mind: Visualizing the Brain from Antiquity to the 21st Century*. Abrams, 2010.
Schroeder, Doris, et al., eds., *Ethics Dumping: Case Studies from North-South Research Collaborations*. Springer Open, 2018.
Schwenk, Thomas L., and Katharine J. Gold, 'Physician Burnout—A Serious Symptom, But of What?', *Journal of the American Medical Association* 320, no. 11 (280): 1109–10.
Scull, Andrew, *Decarceration: Community Treatment and the Deviant—A Radical View*. Prentice-Hall, 1977.
Scull, Andrew, *Hysteria: The Disturbing History*. Oxford University Press, 2012.
Scull, Andrew, 'Madness in the Ancient and Medieval Worlds', in *The Routledge History of Madness and Mental Health*, ed. Greg Eghigian. Routledge, 2017, pp. 17–80.
Scull, Andrew, *Madness in Civilisation: A Cultural History of Insanity from the Bible to Freud, from the Madhouse to Modern Medicine*. Thames and Hudson, 2015.
Scull, Andrew, 'The Mental Health Sector and the Social Sciences in Post-World War II USA. Part 1: Total War and Its Aftermath', *History of Psychiatry* 22, no. 1 (2010): 11–14.
Scull, Andrew, *Museums of Madness: The Social Organization of Insanity in Nineteenth-Century England*. Penguin, 1979.
Scull, Andrew, Nicholas Hervey, and Charlotte MacKenzie, *Masters of Bedlam: The Transformation of the Mad-Doctoring Trade*. Princeton University Press, 2014.
Scull, Andrew, 'Rosenhan Revisited: Successful Scientific Fraud', *History of Psychiatry* 34, no. 2 (2023): 180–95.
Scull, Andrew, 'Somatic Treatments and the Historiography of Psychiatry', *History of Psychiatry* 5, no. 17 (1994): 1–12.
Scull, Andrew, 'UK Deinstitutionalisation: Neoliberal Values and Mental Health', in *Mind, State and Society: Social History of Psychiatry and Mental Health in Britain 1960–2010*, ed. George Ikkos and Nick Bouras. Cambridge University Press, 2021, pp. 306–14.
Sedgwick, Peter, *Psycho Politics*. Verso, 2022 (first published 1982).

Seeman, Mary V., 'History of the Dopamine Hypothesis of Antipsychotic Action', *World Journal of Psychiatry* 11, no. 7 (2021): 355–64.
'Self-Knowledge and Mental Health', *The Lancet* 212, no. 5482 (22 September 1928): 611–12.
Seligman, Martin, 'The Hoffman Report, the Central Intelligence Agency, and the Defense of the Nation: A Personal View', *Health Psychology Open* 5, no. 2 (2018): 8.
Serpico, Davide, 'The Cyclical Return of the IQ Controversy: Revisiting the Lessons of the Resolution on Genetics, Race and Intelligence', *Journal of the History of Biology* 54 (2021): 199–228.
Seth, Suman, 'Colonial History and Postcolonial Science Studies', *Radical History Review* 127 (2017): 76.
Sha, Zhiqiang, et al., 'Common Dysfunction of Large-Scale Neurocognitive Networks Across Psychiatric Disorders', *Biological Psychiatry* 85 (2019): 379–88.
Shapira, Elana, and Daniela Finzi, eds., *Freud and the Émigré: Austrian Émigrés, Exiles and the Legacy of Psychoanalysis in Britain, 1930s—1970s*. Springer, 2020.
Shatan, C.F., 'Post-Vietnam Syndrome', *The New York Times*, 6 May 1972: 35.
Shaw, Clare, and Gillian Proctor, 'Women at the Margins: A Critique of the Diagnosis of Borderline Personality Disorder', *Feminism & Psychology* 15, no. 4 (2005): 483–90.
Shaw, T., et al., 'What Is eHealth (6)? Development of a Conceptual Model for eHealth: Qualitative Study with Key Informants', *Journal of Medical Internet Research* 19, no. 10 (2017): e324.
Shephard, Ben, *A War of Nerves: Soldiers and Psychiatrists in the Twentieth Century*. Harvard University Press, 2001.
Sherman, Elisabeth M.S., 'Neuropsychological Outcomes After Epilepsy Surgery: Systematic Review and Pooled Estimates', *Epilepsia* 52 (2011): 857–69.
Shorter, Edward, 'The History of Lithium Therapy', *Bipolar Disorders* 11 (2009): 4–9.
Shorter, Edward, *A History of Psychiatry: From the Era of the Asylum to the Age of Prozac*. John Wiley & Sons, 1997.
Shorter, Edward, and David Healy, *Shock Therapy: A History of Electroconvulsive Treatment in Mental Illness*. Rutgers University Press, 2007.
Shorvon, Simon D., *The Idea of Epilepsy: A Medical and Social History of Epilepsy in the Modern Era (1860–2020)*. Cambridge University Press, 2023.
Showalter, Elaine, *The Female Malady*. Virago, 1987.
Simmel, Georg, 'The Metropolis and Mental Life', in *The Sociology of Georg Simmel*, ed. Kurt H. Wolff. Free Press, 1950.
Sirotkina, Irina, and Marina Kokorina, 'The Dialectics of Labour in a Psychiatric Ward: Work Therapy in the Kaschenko Hospital', in *Psychiatry in Communist Europe*, ed. Mat Savelli and Sarah Marks. Palgrave Macmillan, 2015, pp. 27–49.
Skorburg, Joshua August, and Phoebe Friesen, 'Mind the Gaps: Ethical and Epistemic Issues in the Digital Mental Health Response to Covid-19', *Hastings Center Report,* 51, no. 6 (2021): 23–26.
Slotkin, R., *Gunfighter Nation: The Myth of the Frontier in Twentieth Century America*. HarperPerennial, 1993.
Smail, Daniel Lord, 'Hoarding and the Human Past', *Isis* 105 (2014): 113.
Smail, Daniel Lord, *On Deep History and the Brain*. University of California Press, 2008.
Smith, Clagett G., and Arnold S. Tannenbaum, 'Organizational Control Structure: A Comparative Analysis', *Human Relations* 16, no. 4 (1963): 299–316.
Smith, Gregory W.H., *Erving Goffman*. Routledge, 2006.
Smith, K., '"A Rather Straightforward Problem": Unravelling Networks of Segregation in Alabama's Psychiatric Hospitals, 1966–1972', in *Viral Networks: Connecting Digital Humanities and Medical History*, ed. E.T. Ewing and K. Randall. Virginia Tech Publishing, 2018, pp. 31–58.
Smith, Leonard, *Private Madhouses in England, 1640–1815: Commercialised Care for the Insane*. Palgrave, 2020.

Smith, Matt, *The First Resort: The History of Social Psychiatry in the United States*. Columbia University Press, 2023.
Socarides, Charles W., 'Homosexuality: Findings Derived from 15 Years of Clinical Research' in R.J. Stoller et al., 'A Symposium: Should Homosexuality Be in the APA Nomenclature?', *American Journal of Psychiatry* 130, no. 11 (1973): 1213.
Sokolowsky, Laura, *Psychoanalysis Under Nazi Occupation*. Routledge, 2021.
Soled, Derek Ross, et al., 'The Case for Health Reparations', *Frontiers in Public Health* 9 (2021): 1–6.
Solomon, Rebecca Z., 'Women in Psychiatry', *American Journal of Psychiatry* 130, no. 10 (1973): 1136–37.
Spandler, Helen, and Sarah Carr, 'Lesbian and Bisexual Women's Experiences of Aversion Therapy in England', *History of the Human Sciences* 35 (2022): 218–36.
Spitzer, Robert L., 'On Pseudoscience in Science, Logic in Remission, and Psychiatric Diagnosis: A Critique of Rosenhan's "On Being Sane in Insane Places"', *Journal of Abnormal Psychology* 84, no. 5 (1975): 442–52.
Stanton, Alfred H., and Morris S. Schwartz, *The Mental Hospital: A Study of Institutional Participation in Psychiatric Illness and Treatment*. Basic Books, 1954.
Stark, Luke, 'Albert Ellis, Rational Therapy and the Media of "Modern" Emotional Management', *History of the Human Sciences* 10 (2017): 54–74.
Staub, Michael E., *The Mismeasure of Minds: Debating Race and Intelligence Between Brown and the Bell Curve*. University of North Carolina Press, 2018.
Strange, R.E., and D.E. Brown, 'Home from the War: A Study of Psychiatric Problems in Viet Nam Returnees', *American Journal of Psychiatry* 127, no. 4 (1970): 488–92.
Straub, Michael, *Madness Is Civilization: When the Diagnosis Was Social, 1948–1980*. University of Chicago Press, 2011.
'A Stroke Stole Her Ability to Speak at 30. A.I. Is Helping to Restore It Years Later', *New York Times*, 23 August 2023, www.nytimes.com/2023/08/23/health/ai-stroke-speech-neuroscience.html.
Sturdy, Steve, Richard Freeman, and Jennifer Smith-Merry, 'Making Knowledge for International Policy: WHO Europe and Mental Health Policy, 1970–2008', *Social History of Medicine* 26, no. 3 (2013): 532–54.
Sulloway, Frank J., *Freud: Biologist of the Mind. Beyond the Psychiatric Legend*. Harvard University Press, 1992.
Sumathipala, Athula, and Buddhika Fernando, 'Ethical Issues in Global Mental Health Trials', in *Global Mental Health Trials*, ed. Graham Thornicroft and Vikram Patel. Oxford University Press, 2015, pp. 123–38.
Suri, J., '*AHR* Forum: The Rise and Fall of an International Counterculture, 1960–1975', *AHR* 114, no. 1 (2009): 45–68.
Suzuki, Akihito, *Madness at Home: The Psychiatrist, the Patient and the Family in England, 1820–60*. University of California Press, 2006.
Swartz, Sally, 'Asylum Case Records: Fact and Fiction', *Rethinking History* 22, no. 3 (2018): 289–301.
Szasz, Thomas, 'Debunking Antipsychiatry: Laing, Law, and Largactil', *Existential Analysis* 19, no. 2 (2008): 316–44.
Taitimu, Melissa, et al., 'Ngā Whakāwhitinga (Standing at the Crossroads): How Māori Understand What Western Psychiatry Calls "Schizophrenia"', *Transcultural Psychiatry* 55, no. 2 (2018): 153–77.
Takabayashi, Akinobu, 'Surviving the Lunacy Act of 1890: English Psychiatrists and Professional Development During the Early Twentieth Century', *Medical History* 61, no. 2 (2017): 246–69.
Tang, Jerry, et al., 'Semantic Reconstruction of Continuous Language from Non-invasive Brain Recordings', *Nature Neuroscience*, 1 May 2023.
Tatzer, Ernst, Werner Maleczek, and Franz Waldhauser, 'An Assessment of What Hans Asperger Knew About Child Euthanasia in Vienna During the Nazi Occupation', *Acta Paediatrica* 112, no. 5 (2023): 1109–19

Taylor, Steven J., *Acts of Conscience: World War II, Mental Institutions, and Religious Objectors*. Syracuse University Press, 2009.
Taylor, Warren D., 'Depression in the Elderly', *New England Journal of Medicine* 371 (2014): 1228–36.
Taylor-Robinson, S.D., et al., 'Why Is There a Paucity of Clinical Trials in Africa?', *QJM: An International Journal of Medicine* 114, no. 6 (2021): 357–58.
Thalassis, Nafiska, 'Soldiers in Psychiatric Therapy: The Case of Northfield Military Hospital 1942–1946', *Social History of Medicine* 20, no. 2 (2007): 351–68.
'This Machine Can Read Your Mind and Translate How You See the World', *BBC Science Focus*, 2 May 2023, www.sciencefocus.com/news/this-machine-can-read-your-mind-and-translate-how-you-see-the-world.
Thomas, Julie Adeney, 'History and Biology in the Anthropocene: Problems of Scale, Problems of Value', *American Historical Review* 119 (2014): 1587–607.
Thomas, K.K., *Deluxe Jim Crow: Civil Rights and American Health Policy, 1935–1954*. University of Georgia Press, 2011.
Thomson, Mathew, 'Mental Hygiene as an International Movement', in *International Health Organisations and Movements, 1918–1939*, ed. Paul Weindling. Cambridge University Press, 1995, pp. 283–304.
Thomson, Mathew, *The Problem of Mental Deficiency: Eugenics, Democracy, and Social Policy in Britain, c.1870–1959*. Oxford University Press, 1998.
Thomson, Mathew, *Psychological Subjects: Identity, Culture, and Health in Twentieth-Century Britain*. Oxford University Press, 2006.
Tiffany, W.J., 'The Mental Health of Army Troops in Viet Nam', *American Journal of Psychiatry* 123, no. 12 (1967): 1585–86.
Tiffany, W.J., and W. Allerton, 'Army Psychiatry in the Mid-60s', *American Journal of Psychiatry* 123, no. 7 (1967): 810–18.
Todes, Daniel P., *Ivan Pavlov: A Russian Life in Science*. Oxford University Press, 2014.
Tomes, Nancy, *A Generous Confidence: Thomas Story Kirkbride and the Art of Asylum Keeping, 1840–1883*. reprinted Cambridge University Press, 2016.
Tomes, Nancy, 'Historical Perspectives on Women and Mental Illness', in *Women, Health, and Medicine in America: A Historical Handbook*, ed. Rima D. Apple. Garland Publishing, 1990, pp. 143–72.
Tomes, Nancy, 'The Patient as a Policy Factor: A Historical Case Study of the Consumer/Survivor Movement in Mental Health', *Health Affairs* (May/June 2006): 720–29.
Topp, Leslie, *Freedom and the Cage: Modern Architecture and Psychiatry in Central Europe, 1890–1914*. Pennsylvania State University Press, 2017.
Torous, John, et al., 'The Growing Field of Digital Psychiatry: Current Evidence and the Future of Apps, Social Media, Chatbots, and Virtual Reality', *World Psychiatry* 20, no. 3 (2021): 318–35.
Treatment Advocacy Center, 'More Mentally Ill Persons Are in Jails and Prisons than Hospitals: A Survey of the States', *Treatment Advocacy Center*, 2010, https://san-mateo.networkofcare.org/library/final_jails_v_hospitals_study1.pdf.
'Treatment of Alcoholics and Drug Addicts in Fraser House Neurosis and Alcoholic Unit, North Ryde Psychiatric Centre', in Neville T. Yeomans Papers, 1960–1971, State Library of New South Wales, MLMSS. 2416/2, Papers re Fraser House, 1960–1967.
Tsou, Jonathan Y., 'Natural Kinds, Psychiatric Classification and the History of the *DSM*', *History of Psychiatry* 27, no. 4 (2016): 406–24.
Tuck, Eve, and K. Wayne Yang, 'Decolonization Is Not a Metaphor', *Decolonization: Indigeneity, Education & Society* 1 (2012): 1–40.
Turda, Marius, 'New Perspectives on Race and Eugenics', *The Historical Journal* 51 (2008): 1115–24.
Turkle, Sherry, *The Second Self: Computers and the Human Spirit*. The MIT Press, 2005.
Turner, John, et al., 'The History of Mental Health Services in Modern England: Practitioner Memories and the Direction of Future Research', *Medical History* 59, no. 4 (2015): 599–624.

Ussher, Jane M., 'The Construction and Lived Experience of Women's Distress: Positioning Premenstrual Change as Psychiatric Illness', in *The Madness of Women: Myth and Experience*. Routledge, 2011, pp. 153–84.

Uzarczyk, Kamila, '"Schluss Mit Der Rassenschande!" From Separation to Extermination: The Fate of Jewish Mentally Ill Patients in Germany and Occupied Poland, 1939–42', in *Recognizing the Past in the Present: New Studies on Medicine Before, During, and After the Holocaust*, ed. Sabine Hildebrandt, Miriam Offer and Michael A. Grodin. Berghahn Books, 2020, pp. 257–75.

van den Oever, Roel, *Mama's Boy: Momism and Homophobia in Postwar American Culture*. Palgrave Macmillan, 2012.

Van Der Kolk, Bessel, *The Body Keeps the Score: Mind, Brain and Body in the Transformation of Trauma*. Penguin, 2014.

Varadarajulu, Rachel, and Ananya Mahapatra, 'Prisoner Mental Health in the United States of America and India: A Dual Perspective', *World Social Psychiatry* 5, no. 1 (2023): 42–46.

Varon, J.P., *Bringing the War Home: The Weather Underground, the Red Army Faction, and Revolutionary Violence in the Sixties and Seventies*. University of California Press, 2004.

Vaughan, Megan, *Curing Their Ills: Colonial Power and African Illness*. Stanford University Press, 1991.

Vicedo, Marga, *The Nature and Nurture of Love: From Imprinting to Attachment in Cold War America*. University of Chicago Press, 2013.

Vidal, Carol, et al., 'Social Media Use and Depression in Adolescents: A Scoping Review', *International Review of Psychiatry* 32, no. 3 (2020): 235.

Volkmann, Constantin, 'Lithium Treatment Over the Lifespan in Bipolar Disorders', *Fronters in Psychiatry* 11 (2020): Article 377, 1–11.

Waddington, Keir, '"Unsuitable Cases": The Debate Over Outpatient Admissions, the Medical Profession and the Late-Victorian London Hospitals', *Medical History* 42 (1998): 26–46.

Waitoki, W., et al., 'Indigenous Psychology in Aotearoa/New Zealand and Australia', in *Global Psychologies: Mental Health and the Global South*, ed. Suman Fernando and Roy Moodley. Palgrave Macmillan, 2018, pp. 163–84.

Wake, Naoko, 'The Military, Psychiatry, and "Unfit" Soldiers, 1939–1942', *Journal of the History of Medicine and Allied Sciences* 62, no. 4 (2007): 461–94.

Wake, Naoko, *Private Practices: Harry Stack Sullivan, the Science of Homosexuality, and American Liberalism*. Rutgers University Press, 2011.

Walkup, James, 'The Psychiatric Unit Comes to the General Hospital: A History of the Movement,' *New Directions for Mental Health Services* 73 (1997): 11–23.

Wall, Oisin, *The British Anti-psychiatrists: From Institutional Psychiatry to the Counter-culture, 1960–1971*. Routledge, 2018.

Wallbridge, D.C., 'Pseudopatients', *British Medical Journal* (8 February 1975): 334.

Waln, Robert, 'An Account of the Asylum for the Insane: Established by the Society of Friends, near Frankford, in the Vicinity of Philadelphia', *Philadelphia Journal of the Medical and Physical Sciences* (August 1825): 15.

Walsh, R.J., 'Experimental Pseudopatients', *Medical Journal of Australia* (8 June 1974): 944.

Waltraud, Ernst, *Mad Tales from the Raj: Colonial Psychiatry in South Asia, 1800–58*. Anthem Press, 2010.

Waltraud, Ernst, ed., *Work, Psychiatry and Society, c.1750–2015*. Manchester University Press, 2016.

Warr, Deborah, et al., 'Hype, Evidence Gaps and Digital Divides: Telehealth Blind Spots in Rural Australia', *Health: An Interdisciplinary Journal for the Social Study of Health, Illness and Medicine* 27 (2021): 588–606.

Warsh, Cheryl Krasnick, and Veronica Strong-Boag, eds., *Children's Health Issues in Historical Perspective*. Wilfrid Laurier University Press, 2005.

Webb, Christian A., et al., 'Personalized Prediction of Antidepressant *v.* Placebo Response: Evidence from the EMBARC Study', *Psychological Medicine* 49 (2019): 1118–27.

Weber, Max, *The Protestant Ethic and the Spirit of Capitalism*, trans. Talcott Parsons. Routledge, 2001.

Weindling, Paul, et al., 'The Problematic Legacy of Victim Specimens from the Nazi Era: Identifying the Persons Behind the Specimens at the Max Planck Institutes for Brain Research and of Psychiatry', *Journal of the History of the Neurosciences* 32, no. 2 (2023): 218–39.

Weiner, Dora B., 'Mind and Body in the Clinic: Philippe Pinel, Alexander Crichton, Dominique Esquirol, and the Birth of Psychiatry', in *The Languages of Psyche: Mind and Body in Enlightenment Thought*, ed. G.S. Rousseau. University of California Press, 1990, pp. 331–402.

Weizenbaum, Joseph, 'Computers as "Therapists"', *Science* 198, no. 4315 (1977): 354.

Weizenbaum, Joseph, 'ELIZA—A Computer Program for the Study of Natural Language Communication Between Man and Machine', *Communications of the ACM* 9, no. 1 (1966): 36–45.

Welch, Steven R., 'Military Justice', in *1914–1918 Online: International Encyclopedia of the First World War*, 2014, https://encyclopedia.1914-1918-online.net/article/military_justice.

Werkhoven, Sander, 'Natural Kinds of Mental Disorder', *Synthese* 199 (2021): 10135–65.

West, Louis Jolyon, et al., 'An Approach to the Problem of Homosexuals in the Military Service', *American Journal of Psychiatry* 115, no. 5 (1958): 392–401.

Westbury, Juanita, et al., 'More Action Needed: Psychotropic Prescribing in Australian Residential Aged Care', *Australian and New Zealand Journal of Psychiatry* 53, no. 2 (2019): 136–47.

Wexler, Lisa, et al., 'Advancing Suicide Prevention Research with Rural American Indian and Alaska Native Populations', *American Journal of Public Health* 105, no. 5 (2014): 891–99.

Wheatland, Thomas, *The Frankfurt School in Exile*. University of Minnesota Press, 2009.

Wild, Georgina, et al., 'The Penrose Hypothesis in the Second Half of the 20th Century: Investigating the Relationship Between Psychiatric Bed Numbers and the Prison Population in England Between 1960 and 2018–2019', *British Journal of Psychiatry* 220, no. 5 (2022): 295–301.

Williams, S.C.P., 'Epigenetics', *PNAS* 110 (2013): 3209.

Wilson, Elizabeth A., *Affect and Artificial Intelligence*. University of Washington Press, 2010.

Wing, J.K., and G.W. Brown, *Institutionalism and Schizophrenia: A Comparative Study of Three Mental Hospitals*. Cambridge University Press, 1970.

Winkler, Robin C., 'Research into Mental Health Practice Using Pseudopatients', *Medical Journal of Australia* 2 (14 September 1974): 399–403.

Winkler, Rolfe, 'The Failed Promise of Online Mental-health Treatment', *Wall Street Journal* (19 December 2022). www.wsj.com/articles/the-failed-promise-of-online-mental-health-treatment-11671390353.

Wolfe, Charles T., 'Introduction', in *Brain Theory: Essays in Critical Neurophilosophy*. Palgrave, 2014, pp. 1–13.

Woods, Angela, *The Sublime Object of Psychiatry: Schizophrenia in Clinical and Cultural Theory*. Oxford University Press, 2011.

Woods, Angela, 'Voices, Identity, and Meaning-making', *The Lancet* (12 December 2015): 2386–87.

Woods, Randall B., *Prisoners of Hope: Lyndon B. Johnson, the Great Society, and the Limits of Liberalism*. Basic Books, 2016.

World Federation for Mental Health, *Mental Health and World Citizenship: A Statement Prepared for the International Congress on Mental Health*. World Federation for Mental Health, 1948.

World Health Organization, *WHO and Mental Health, 1949–1961*. World Health Organization, 1962.
Wright, David, *Mental Disability in Victorian England: The Earlswood Asylum 1847–1901*. Oxford University Press, 2001.
Wright, David, 'Re-placing the Lunatic Asylum in the History of Madness', *History Australia* 19, no. 1 (2022): 161–76.
Wu, Harry, *Mad by the Millions*. The MIT Press, 2021.
Yager, J., 'Personal Violence in Infantry Combat', *Archives of General Psychiatry* 32, no. 2 (1975): 257–61.
Yager, J., 'Postcombat Violent Behaviour in Psychiatrically Maladjusting Soldiers', *Archives of General Psychiatry* 33, no. 11 (1976): 1332–35.
Yanni, Carla, *The Architecture of Madness: Insane Asylums in the United States*. University of Minnesota Press, 2007.
Yarbrough, Eric, 'The Gender Dysphoria Diagnosis', in *Transgender Mental Health*. American Psychiatric Association Publishing, 2018, pp. 91–110.
Yehuda, Rachel, and Amy Lehrner, 'Intergenerational Transmission of Trauma Effects: Putative Role of Epigenetic Mechanisms', *World Psychiatry* 17, no. 3 (2018): 243–57.
Young, Alan, *The Harmony of Illusions: Inventing Post-Traumatic Stress Disorder*. Princeton University Press, 1995.
Yuan, Y., et al., 'Use of Antidepressants in U.S. Nursing Home Residents: A Systematic Review', *Innovation in Aging* 2, Suppl 1 (2018): 514.
Zajicek, Benjamin, 'The Psychopharmacological Revolution in the USSR: Schizophrenia Treatment and the Thaw in Soviet Psychiatry, 1954–64', *Medical History* 63, no. 3 (2019): 249–69.
Zajicek, Benjamin, 'Scientific Psychiatry in Stalin's Soviet Union: The Politics of Modern Medicine and the Struggle to Define "Pavlovian" Psychiatry, 1939–1953', PhD thesis, University of Chicago, 2009.
Zajicek, Benjamin, et al., 'Soviet Psychiatry and the Origins of the Sluggish Schizophrenia Concept, 1912–1936', *History of the Human Sciences* 31, no. 2 (2018): 88–105.
Zweiniger-Bargielowska, Ina. *Managing the Body: Beauty, Health and Fitness in Britain, 1880–1939*. Oxford University Press, 2010.

INDEX

FSC
www.fsc.org
MIX
Papier | Fördert
gute Waldnutzung
FSC® C083411

Kolibri 360 GmbH
Ferdinand-Jühlke-Straße 7
99095 Erfurt, Deutschland
produktsicherheit@kolibri360.de